WHAT IF IT'S *NOT* DEPRESSION?

YOUR GUIDE TO FINDING ANSWERS AND SOLUTIONS

ACHINA P. STEIN DO, IFMCP

Advance Praise

"Finally, a book to help the millions of people who have been suffering without getting solid solutions for their woes. This book is so needed, not only for regular people who are seeking answers regarding how to heal their anguish from depression and anxiety, but for the conventional medical community that currently seems to ignore that there are actually true cures for mental illness. In her brilliantly written book, Dr. Achina Stein puts a stop to the Band-Aid approach of putting depression suffers all in the same box and sprinkling them with drugs, which we have long known does not work for many people or long term. As a physician who has been through severe clinical depression and healed naturally with the help of dedicated professionals like Dr. Stein who presented me real solutions that resulted in a complete cure, it makes my heart sing with joy that Dr. Stein is brave enough to publish the path to answers and a possible cure. This is a must read for everyone with any kind of mental illness."

– Veronica Anderson, MD, author of Too Smart to Be Struggling: The Guide for Over-Scheduled Doctors to Find Happiness (and Make More Money, Too)

"This book is gold for people suffering on the psychiatric medication hamster wheel. Dr. Stein uses wonderful analogies and stories and up-to-date science to explain to readers why conventional psychiatry has not been able to help them. She then expertly leads the reader to and through the paradigm shift that must occur in the patient for them to understand how to achieve true healing."

– John Bartemus, DC, BCIM, CFMP

"Dr. Stein does a great job of combining her own personal story and clinical experiences with a commonsense approach to addressing symptoms, namely searching for and trying to understand their underlying causes. Lifestyle changes like diet, meditation, getting enough sleep, and exercise can prevent, reduce, and eliminate many painful symptoms. Clearly-written, engaging, and easy to understand with many practical tools, apps, and references, Dr. Stein's book hits this one out of the park."

– Marshall Wold MD

"Dr. Stein has done a wonderful job showing us what I have found over and over in my Functional Psychiatry practice: depression happens for a variety of reasons, and usually not just one reason.

Following Dr. Stein's useful and insightful advice will undoubtedly be of benefit to you or your loved ones on your healing journey."

– Kat Toups, MD, DFAPA, IFMCP,
author of Dementia Demystified

"I was intrigued and moved by Dr. Stein's narrative. It encourages the reader to think differently about the quality of their

Advance Praise

"Finally, a book to help the millions of people who have been suffering without getting solid solutions for their woes. This book is so needed, not only for regular people who are seeking answers regarding how to heal their anguish from depression and anxiety, but for the conventional medical community that currently seems to ignore that there are actually true cures for mental illness. In her brilliantly written book, Dr. Achina Stein puts a stop to the Band-Aid approach of putting depression suffers all in the same box and sprinkling them with drugs, which we have long known does not work for many people or long term. As a physician who has been through severe clinical depression and healed naturally with the help of dedicated professionals like Dr. Stein who presented me real solutions that resulted in a complete cure, it makes my heart sing with joy that Dr. Stein is brave enough to publish the path to answers and a possible cure. This is a must read for everyone with any kind of mental illness."

– Veronica Anderson, MD, author of Too Smart to Be Struggling: The Guide for Over-Scheduled Doctors to Find Happiness (and Make More Money, Too)

"This book is gold for people suffering on the psychiatric medication hamster wheel. Dr. Stein uses wonderful analogies and stories and up-to-date science to explain to readers why conventional psychiatry has not been able to help them. She then expertly leads the reader to and through the paradigm shift that must occur in the patient for them to understand how to achieve true healing."

– John Bartemus, DC, BCIM, CFMP

"Dr. Stein does a great job of combining her own personal story and clinical experiences with a commonsense approach to addressing symptoms, namely searching for and trying to understand their underlying causes. Lifestyle changes like diet, meditation, getting enough sleep, and exercise can prevent, reduce, and eliminate many painful symptoms. Clearly-written, engaging, and easy to understand with many practical tools, apps, and references, Dr. Stein's book hits this one out of the park."

– Marshall Wold MD

"Dr. Stein has done a wonderful job showing us what I have found over and over in my Functional Psychiatry practice: depression happens for a variety of reasons, and usually not just one reason.

Following Dr. Stein's useful and insightful advice will undoubtedly be of benefit to you or your loved ones on your healing journey."

– Kat Toups, MD, DFAPA, IFMCP,
author of Dementia Demystified

"I was intrigued and moved by Dr. Stein's narrative. It encourages the reader to think differently about the quality of their life and the means to achieve it. It is not only informative but beautifully written."

– Susan Bartolone, EdD

"What If It's NOT Depression?: Your Guide to Solutions and Answers is a long-awaited practical book taking a long-needed look at depression. It speaks to our inner knowing, what we know to be true. Depression diagnosis is a lazy diagnosis, as when you work with humans you discover as you get to know them that there are many causes, masked as depression, that are not appropriately treated with psychotropics. Bravo!"

– Daniel Rieders, MD FACC FHRS CCDS IFMCP

"A must read if you are fatigued or simply don't feel well, have been told your labs are normal and that you are depressed, but in your heart of hearts know that you are not depressed. Dr. Stein is a leader in her industry in regaining optimal health, marrying the fields of traditional medicine, functional medicine, and psychotherapy. A true healer."

– Rajka Milanovic Galbraith, MD IFMCP

This book is dedicated to my mother,
Prafulla (Bandodkar) Palanki.

She is my guardian angel.

She provides me in spirit what she was
unable to provide me when alive.

I wish I could turn back time and
use the knowledge I have now to
give her the life she deserved.

Contents

Foreword

More than 60 million Americans–that's about one in four–are affected by mental health issues every year. Rather than determine what might actually be causing that depression, many doctors immediately reach for their prescription pads. That explains why one in ten Americans today uses antidepressants.

While drugs can be lifesaving in some cases, many people have poor or suboptimal results and/or severe side effects. They aren't given many other choices. Conventional medicine fails to address the underlying causes of what might seem like depression and why they differ from one person to another. Instead, they label the disease and approach the treatment identically – even though the cause of that disease may be radically different from person to person. Ultimately, drugs like antidepressants don't cure the disease, they just mask the symptoms.

As a functional medicine doctor, I take a different approach to depression by trying to understand what creates it. To call someone depressed says nothing about the underlying causes that create depression. I believe the key to this new paradigm is this: depression is not in our heads. It is in our bodies. When we fix the body, we fix the brain. Our energy, memory, focus, and joy all increase, and depression will likely fade away.

While simple, this approach requires digging deep and connecting patterns. Dr. Achina Stein's new book, *What If It's Not Depression?: Your Guide to Answers and Solutions* is a lifeline to patients in just this situation. Dr. Stein shares the benefit of over twenty-five years of experience treating depression in a variety of clinical settings: community mental health centers, hospitals, private practice, and the prison system. She helps readers understand *why* they may have received a diagnosis of depression from a conventional doctor and what this diagnosis really means. Among the most compelling chapters of the book is Dr. Stein's sharing of her own discovery of functional medicine while searching for answers to health problems in her immediate family. Despite being a practicing psychiatrist, she found herself at a loss when confronted with her own children's mental health issues. She had the experience to know the limitations of standard psychiatric care and intuitively felt that there must be a better way.

Dr. Stein guides readers step-by-step through a functional medicine approach to discovering the root causes of symptoms. In truth, many depressive symptoms have their origin in the gut, as about seventy percent of the immune system is in the gut lining. Disruptions from healthy gut functioning including microbes, environmental toxins, allergens, stress, and poor diet cause inflammation and produce both physical and mental effects. Dr. Stein invites readers to be "Sherlock Holmes" searching for clues to their physical and mental health challenges. As a classically-trained psychiatrist, she was experienced in using the psychodynamic and biopsychosocial approach as tools for parsing out the layers of multiple root causes emotionally, but as a functional medicine practitioner, she used those same skills to parse the layers out physically.

She guides readers through the development of their own medical timelines and provides detailed information on their use and importance. She shows how the different systems within the body are like an orchestra playing a piece of music.

Dr. Stein leads the reader from diagnosis to action through a paradigm SHIFT of their physiology. SHIFT is a good acronym for the bad actors that she is helping readers remove: stress, hormones, infections, foods, and toxins. By removing these, readers will reduce inflammation and put out the metaphorical fire so that the body can start repairing. In every chapter the book contains practical diagnostic tools and a plan for action. The diet and lifestyle changes Dr. Stein leads the reader through are often hard work requiring patience, self-discipline, and perseverance.

Dr. Stein's specialization in psychiatry and her many years of clinical psychiatric experience give her a unique perspective. As the co-founder of Functional Mind, LLC in 2016, she has improved the lives of many patients with mental health issues. The approach of finding and removing multiple root causes of chronic depression and supporting gut health through supplements and dietary and lifestyle changes is at the cutting edge of medicine. Although antidepressants are unquestionably the right call for certain patients and in acute situations, Dr. Stein has been helping patients achieve lasting results and avoid or even taper off medications, if warranted.

This book not only guides readers to the answer of the title question, *What if It's Not Depression?*, it then explains what the reader can do about it. It provides hope through a functional medical approach that there might be alternatives to taking medications long term or at all.

Dr. Mark Hyman

https://drhyman.com/

Introduction

Katie is a powerhouse and has been driving herself through everything she has to do for the past two years. She works full time at a museum and, with her husband, raises two children. She's fortunate to have a modern husband who cooks and cleans. He is so supportive of her. Her kids are pre-teens and she is not looking forward to their hormonal changes. She's got enough to handle between managing the museum, her house, and the estate of her late brother.

He died of brain cancer a year ago, but she still has been dealing with the estate. She's always been the peacemaker and the caregiver of the family. Her parents aren't able to deal with any of this stuff so, naturally, it falls on her. She doesn't think she's even had time to deal with the loss. She has two other brothers, but they live far away. Even if they lived close by, they would likely have been more of a hindrance than a help. They have their own families and it's easier for Katie to just take care of things herself.

The year before her brother died took a toll on her. She had been actively going to the gym and yoga classes, but those things slowly dropped off and she hasn't been able to get them back into her routine. She's just exhausted by the end of the day. She's always liked coffee in the morning; it's part of her morning ritual with her husband once the kids are on the bus. But she's been drinking another cup of coffee to get herself moving recently and lately has even started to have another cup in the afternoon around three or four p.m. She's got a long to-do list and prides herself on being super organized, but lately she just doesn't have the energy.

Sometimes, she stays late at work. She always hated having loose ends at the end of the day and likes to leave the office on time with all of her to-dos crossed off. Lately, she has become less efficient, leaving things unfinished, and is forced to leave the office to get the kids from their activities and start dinner. She is constantly juggling. Now she finds herself having trouble falling asleep because she's thinking about all the things she needs to do and how she is going to do them the next day. Every so often, some sadness creeps in about her brother. *I really miss him*, she thinks.

She starts to have a glass of wine every night after dinner, which turns into two glasses. Red wine is good for you; she read that in some magazine. After a meal, she starts to get some bloating, gas, and acne breakouts. She used to get headaches rarely, but now they are about once a week.

Her boss calls her into her office and says that she hasn't been on the ball. People are noticing that she's a little spaced out. She admits to having some brain fog and not being able to concentrate. Her boss had been understanding about the loss of her brother, but that was a year ago.

What's going on now? Katie asks herself. *What's wrong with me?*

A good friend of hers felt the same way, almost to a T. That friend went to the doctor, who ran some testing and found out she had a thyroid problem. Maybe that's what's going on.

Katie Googled fatigue and read about low iron. Maybe she has that? Another one of her friends did because she had really heavy periods. *But I don't have heavy periods.* Katie decides to call her doctor. The last time she went to the doctor was for a UTI, and the time before that was for her annual physical exam. Her doctor orders her some blood work and a urinalysis.

She likes her doctor but hates going to the office. There are too many sick people. She prefers to wait outside in the sunshine. The receptionist knows where to find her. The doctor does a cursory exam and asks her some questions she doesn't feel are relevant, but oh well. The doctor is just doing her job. The doctor tells her that her blood work is normal and there is nothing wrong medically. She brings up the fact that Katie's brother died and that perhaps she might be depressed. Stunned by this, Katie doesn't register everything that follows.

She walks out of the office with a prescription for an antidepressant. She looks at it and thinks, *Am I depressed?* She feels like this is a life sentence. She has friends on antidepressants. They never really talk about why. She sees the commercials on TV but never thought they applied to her. Then she thinks, *Is what I'm feeling what they're talking about?* She considers different family members and remembers Uncle Joe, who was depressed and had PTSD when he came back from WWII. She had heard stories of a distant aunt who was a recluse. Her brothers are both irritable, so maybe this is just normal for her family. Now she is having doubts and second-guessing herself. *I guess I don't have much choice. Or do I? I wish I had more time with my doctor to discuss other options. You can't talk about much in fifteen minutes. She just keeps telling me to slow down.*

Katie tries the antidepressant for a week. It causes her to become very anxious and nauseous, and it irritates her stomach. Her doctor warned her about that. She stops the antidepressant and goes back to her doctor to find out what else can be done. Katie tries to explain that other things are going on in her body that just aren't right and asks for further testing. She tells her doctor that she Googled causes of fatigue and that maybe she has low iron. She has a fleeting thought that maybe she has cancer and it hasn't been detected yet. It took so long for her brother to figure out that he had cancer.

Her doctor rolls her eyes and says, "Your blood work is normal. There is no evidence of cancer and no need to do further blood work." She recommends that Katie see a psychiatrist because she needs to be evaluated for another antidepressant and provides a couple of names. "You're telling me I'm crazy?" Katie asks. The doctor looks at her watch and gets up to leave, saying, "No, I'm not saying you're crazy. I don't really know what else to do. Maybe seeing a psychotherapist will help you sort things out. You can pick up a list of psychotherapists we refer to at the front desk."

Does this sound familiar?

CHAPTER 1

Last Stop on the Crazy Train!

Most of the people I work with have had Katie's experience or worse. Many feel they actually have a good relationship with their doctors, but they want more of their time. One childhood friend of mine was psychiatrically hospitalized because she said she would kill herself if someone didn't help her with her debilitating physical symptoms. She was at the end of her rope. She went to multiple doctors, chiropractors, and pain specialists. Ultimately, she was told that she was a hypochondriac because she suggested that she thought that she might have cancer. She reached out to me for help. After several hours of just listening to her story in detail, I was able to tell her she had a pelvic subluxation that was causing her pain and directed her to an osteopathic physician in her area to confirm this, ultimately resolving the problem. She experienced relief within a day of the first treatment. Most importantly, she received confirmation that she wasn't losing her mind and that she, indeed, does not have cancer.

Some of my patients have been to multiple specialists and psychiatrists to try to figure out what's wrong with them. Being referred to a psychiatrist is a double-edged sword. Maybe you do need to see a psychiatrist, and they will confirm that. Many psychiatrists rarely tell a patient that they don't have a psychiatric problem once they are referred and seen in the office. It's almost like they forget what normal is. They are even less likely to do a detailed physical history, exam, or workup to rule out a physical cause beyond the most basic testing. They assume that the primary care physician (PCP) did their due diligence and ruled out all physical (also known as "medical") causes and wouldn't have made the referral if it wasn't warranted. Most psychiatrists approach a patient from that vantage point.

Regardless, the only options typically offered are medications and psychotherapy. Often, the first cut of psychiatry is to "match the pill to the ill." Psychiatrists do less and less psychotherapy as compared to two or three decades ago. Today psychiatrists typically do an hour-long initial evaluation using a decision tree to document all of a patient's psychiatric symptoms and rule out possibilities to finally arrive at a diagnosis. For the most part, that's the whole process – to match a medication to the diagnosis. The alternate purposes of diagnoses are for identifying participants for potential research, conveying information between clinicians, and billing insurance companies.

The idea that depression results from a chemical imbalance in the brain was first proposed in the late 1950s and early 1960s by several scientists. The focus was initially on the neurotransmitter norepinephrine. However, by the mid-1960s the focus had shifted to serotonin, another neurotransmitter, which led to the development of Selective Serotonin Reuptake Inhibitors (SSRI) such as Prozac and Paxil. Dopamine is a third type of neurotransmitter that can affect the mood. Patients embraced this theory because it was better than being told they had a character flaw; it was an explanation that settled better. They could now say, "It's not my fault." NAMI (National Alliance on Mental Illness) embraced this theory and promoted it. Lives have been saved and/or improved with medications. But did you know that the chemical imbalance theory has been largely discredited?

We don't know why these antidepressant medications work. Yet we still prescribe them. Why? Because they work for some people for some of the time. When there is an emergency, there really isn't anything else to offer. They don't help everyone, and they do cause many side effects. Some people have serious withdrawal symptoms.

Research is now showing that the long-term benefits from medications may not outweigh the increased risk of heart attacks, strokes, and diabetes. The American Psychiatric Association (APA) does not denounce the long-term use of antidepressant medications despite mounting evidence of ineffectiveness over time, and lack of research to support their use beyond two years. There is no disease that is being treated (which I'll explain below). No scan for depression. No blood testing. When you look at *all* of the research on antidepressant medication, the results of medications are slightly better than placebo but clinically insignificant.

Medications did solve a problem. And they still do...for some. I've worked at the Bridgewater State Hospital – moonlighting on the weekends. It's one of two hospitals in the country that have inmates with serious psychiatric illnesses. From time to time, a patient there might refuse to take medication and become floridly psychotic. They become very sick, for weeks sometimes, in their own living hell until a court order is received allowing a psychiatrist to provide medication against the patient's will. And within days, the patient is lucid again. There really is no other solution for this population.

However, on the other extreme it is quite outrageous that we are giving five-year-old children anti-psychotic medication for behavioral disorders. Yes, there might be that one instance that a five-year-old needs it, after careful consideration and as a last resort. But there are far too many five-year-olds on psychotropic medication. There are more and more children with ADD, ADHD, OCD, major depression, bipolar disorder, and the list goes on.

So how did we get here? Let me lay out the history…

The first systematic study of mental illness occurred in 1840, when the census recorded the frequency of "idiocy and insanity." That's right, mental illness wasn't studied systematically until two hundred years ago. By the 1880 census, seven categories of mental health were distinguished: mania, melancholia, monomania, paresis, dementia, dipsomania, and epilepsy.

In 1917, the American Medico-Psychological Association (now known as the American Psychiatric Association, or APA) began gathering uniform health statistics across mental hospitals for administrative classification reasons. This group created the first psychiatric diagnostic manual.

In 1952, the first edition of the Diagnostic and Statistical Manual, or DSM, was published. The DSM-I contained a glossary of descriptions of the diagnostic categories and was the first official manual of mental disorders to focus on clinical use. The use of the term "reaction" throughout DSM reflected the influence of Adolf Meyer's psychobiological view that "mental disorders represented reactions of the personality to psychological, social, and biological factors." The next edition, DSM-II, was similar to DSM but eliminated the term "reaction."

According to some accounts, in the late 1970s, psychiatry as a profession was criticized for being a less than legitimate field, so the biomedical model of mental disorders was created, as that model would naturally emphasize the importance of taking "medications" for what then became diseases – and it was only psychiatrists who could prescribe those medications. As if psychiatrists are no different than cardiologists! This started with the publication of the DSM-III in 1980, which introduced a number of important innovations, including explicit diagnostic criteria, a multiaxial diagnostic assessment system, and an approach that attempted to be "neutral with respect to the *causes* of mental disorders." It was at this point the search for causes went to the wayside, because there was the belief that medications would resolve all symptoms, and the only thing necessary was to keep tweaking medications until you found the right doses and combinations to put the symptoms in remission. Born were the psychopharmacologists and the problems with polypharmacy.

The most recent edition of the DSM, DSM-5, was published in 2013, adding even more diagnoses. These were sincere efforts by thoughtful professionals to try to make diagnoses more systematic, but in the end, the hyper-classification had missed the point. Generating more labels still focused on the *what*, not the *why*. For example, childhood trauma is nowhere in the DSM. This is a major cause of symptoms, which may be expressed in a myriad of diagnoses, sometimes as many as five! The closest thing that was proposed for the DSM-5, but not accepted was Developmental Trauma Disorder by Bessel van der Kolk, M.D. who wrote *The Body Keeps the Score*. It's not clear to me why this is the case, but I suspect it's because we've set up a medical system to make quick decisions to match a pill to an ill. Knowing that someone has trauma doesn't lead to the proper choice of medications, diagnoses do. I feel the opposite is worse. Focusing on symptoms can overlook trauma and prevent an appropriate referral to a psychotherapist.

Now it seems we pathologize grief, sadness, mid-life, and existential crises so that physicians can have something at hand to offer patients. Unfortunately, these "diagnoses" now feel like life sentences for some people; as if it was something they were born with and can't fix. They fear they will be relegated to taking medications for the rest of their lives and that it will likely be a persistent and chronic downward spiral. That's not very empowering, is it?

By the way, there is little evidence that any of these "disorders" are genetic. Just because something runs in the family doesn't make it genetic. There is a whole new field, epigenetics, the study of biological mechanisms that will switch genes on and off, which is showing promise. The field of epigenetics is quickly growing and with it the understanding that both the environment and individual lifestyle can directly interact with the genome to influence epigenetic change. These changes may be reflected at various stages throughout a person's life and even in later generations. For example, human epidemiological studies have provided evidence that prenatal and early postnatal environmental factors influence the adult risk of developing various chronic diseases and behavioral disorders, like depression.

My preference is to use the words "mental distress" when I see patients because it doesn't presume that they even understand what they are experiencing, and it also doesn't presume that it's a disease or disorder. My assessment starts with a blank slate. It starts with asking a patient what they are experiencing without the psychobabble. Have you ever heard someone say, "I had a manic episode," or 'I had a panic attack" but when you really get down to what they experienced, it wasn't actually a panic attack or manic episode? A modern phenomenon – Dr. Google damage.

The path of healing starts with a blank slate. It starts without assumptions. It starts without judgment. It starts with connecting, helping patients feel safe, heard, and understood. Often with this approach, the healing begins right away.

After psychiatrists prescribe a new medication, they typically have a fifteen-minute follow-up visit about a week after a patient begins the course of treatment. This visit is scheduled to make sure the medication is working, that the benefits outweigh the risks, and to document your history and your informed consent to take the medications. Most follow-up visits beyond that one to six months later are just to do a medication check. Their job is done.

In that informed consent, they don't tell you that the diagnosis they provide is only based on symptoms that you list and not causes. That diagnosis is only as good as the questions they ask and the information you provide. Keeping out one detail can dramatically change that diagnosis. They don't tell you that a record of a psychiatric diagnosis may prevent you from getting into the military, potentially raise your health insurance rates, and/or prevent you from getting disability insurance. Sometimes those conversations don't happen because the benefit highly outweighs the risks and the decision is a "no brainer." Other times antidepressants are handed out like candy.

Many psychiatrists are not comfortable with talking about what is happening in the body. Some psychiatrists do psychotherapy but, again, even then they rarely talk about what is going on in the body. Fewer and fewer graduating psychiatrists these days are required to be trained in psychotherapy, an excellent skill to learn to compassionately discern what a person is experiencing even for diagnostic purposes, if not for treatment as well. I consider this change as a disservice to the field of psychiatry; Sigmund Freud and Carl Jung would roll over in their graves.

How can you see a patient and completely ignore the body? It's attached, isn't it? The head doesn't come boppin' into the office! Yes, psychiatrists do get a past medical and surgical history as part of their initial evaluation, but they rarely delve into it because that's not their area of expertise.

The irony is that psychiatrists are still doctors and are trained as physicians first, so they should be able to do physical exams on their patients and be the ones to determine whether or not a person has something going on in their body that might be the cause of their mental distress. Beyond the basics, the psychiatrist is not trained to do that, nor is the PCP. When a patient has multiple medical and psychiatric issues, there is often a battle over who is responsible. Sometimes patients are ping-ponged back and forth between the medical side and the psychiatric side because no one knows what to do. There are attempts to collaborate through consultation, but it is still siloed assessment and treatment. Doctors don't cross over into another doctor's territory, so to speak. Generally, there is no one overseeing how it's all connected. In the end, a thorough medical workup goes to the wayside.

As a result, the art of medicine is lost. The physical exam, a real thorough physical exam, went out the window when doctors relied mostly on testing. Some doctors never touch their patients...ever. Psychiatrists have been told for years that they shouldn't ever touch their patients. Fortunately, at least for doctors of osteopathy (DOs), like myself, this thinking has changed. The need for a physical exam varies from patient to patient, but it offers clues to what might be going on in the body as a whole. I may do a physical exam if I want to confirm my suspicions about a possible cause or to rule out serious conditions.

Medications can save lives, but they can also wreck them or delay real answers. Some people benefit – the meds work for them and they experience no side effects. They take them for years and do great! It is good fortune to be one of them. Some people take antidepressants, and they work for a month or two, and then stop working so the dose is increased, and they do great! This is also good fortune. Some people are started on antidepressants and they don't work, are switched to another antidepressant, and they still don't work. Others are started on an antidepressant that works well but may have troublesome or intolerable side effects. They might be started on a second medication to deal with the side effects or be put on an adjunct medication to boost the original antidepressant. Suddenly, a patient might be on three medications and feel a little better, but still not be quite right. Something is still off.

It feels like the pharmaceutical industry and insurance industry have hijacked the field of medicine and are telling us how to practice, and we as physicians have let them respectively narrow our treatment options and shorten our sessions. We need to go back to basics – the doctor-patient relationship – and start from scratch.

Other than questions about stressors, something that might explain why, nowhere in this process is there a discovery of *why?* Why is this happening and *why now?*

The point is that every single person should be treated as an individual with a full understanding of all of their problems and how the mind and body are connected. Most chronic problems require many interventions to effect a positive change.

The decision to take medication should be fully informed with a robust discussion about the pros and cons. We are depriving ourselves of the wisdom of the body and mind by applying linear principles to a nonlinear system. All other evidence-based treatment modalities should be discussed in equal parts, but a treatment ought not be discounted just because there isn't a randomized controlled trial or meta-analysis to support it. And finally, a patient's preferences should be part of the decision-making process.

Trust your gut. If you truly believe you are not depressed, start looking for someone who can spend the time with you to sort it out and look for alternative approaches. That's where functional psychiatry comes in. I'm the last stop on the crazy train.

CHAPTER 2

My Story

My mother and I came to the US when I was almost two years old. I was born in India. As the story goes, when my father married my mother, as part of his dowry he was given a promise that he would be educated at a graduate school in the US. He left soon after the wedding, and I didn't meet him until we arrived in the States. My sister was born nine months later. My mother attended night school to learn English. She had an eighth-grade education as that's all that was allowed in her day and age. She had excellent skills as a seamstress and embroidery was her specialty. She was quite industrious as a young woman who helped raise four nieces in Goa, India. She was very smart in her own right and very compassionate.

One night, on her way to night school, my mother was crossing the street in the dark and was hit by a car. She had a significant injury to her head and her knee, and she spent some time in the hospital recovering. What happened six months later has forever been seared into my mind. I was four years old. I was playing with my toys while she started talking to the wall, and then she opened the front door and left. We lived on the sixth floor of an apartment complex, so I went after her. "Mommy, where are you going?" She wouldn't answer and just stared off into the distance. She got into the elevator, and I followed. She went outside, and I followed, this time pulling at her sari, the traditional Indian garment. I remember the day vividly. It was November, very cold outside, and the day was bright and sunny. The leaves were swirling like miniature dust devils, and to this day they remind me of her, and I feel her presence. I was freezing and my teeth were chattering, but I wouldn't let go of her and tried to drag her back. The manager of the building came out and brought us inside. He must have heard me screaming. He wrapped a blanket around me and my mother, then called my father. My mother was taken to an asylum and was there for six months. Later, I was told that she began to have sleep difficulties and started hearing voices telling her that she was a bad wife and a bad mother. She had command hallucinations telling her to go back to India.

When she returned from the hospital, she was somewhat functional but continued to hear voices keeping her up all night for the rest of her life. She was never hospitalized again though. Years later, I realized that she should have been on a higher dose of haloperidol, but perhaps that was the best they could do in the 1960s. Maybe she had intolerable side effects. I'll never know. Nevertheless, she deteriorated, not because of the hallucinations and sleep problems, but because of joint pain. Despite her disability, she managed to have two more children because my father insisted on having sons. To say the least, he was not a kind man. The joint pain worsened and she developed rheumatoid arthritis, which became very severe. Her hands became deformed. She had many treatments, even tried gold injections. Depression set in but not in the classic sense. She couldn't function. By the time I was eight, I was changing my brother's diapers and by eleven, I was running the entire household – balancing the checkbook and raising my three siblings.

When I was sixteen, we went to India during the three-month summer vacation. My siblings had never been there. While we were there, my mother improved – dramatically. It was a wonder. She had no pain, the voices were gone, and she was sleeping! She was happy, talkative, and clearer in her thinking and communication than I had witnessed at any other time. The only thing it didn't change was the deformities of her hands. I told her that she should stay in India. Clearly it was better for her, but she insisted that her home was in the US and she couldn't wait to return, because she missed her soap operas! I didn't believe her. I presumed it was purely psychological and she was in denial.

When we did return to the US, all her symptoms returned with a vengeance.

I went to Rutgers University in New Jersey and studied biology with a specialty in neural science and behavior and received high honors, then went to medical school. I wanted to bring my mother's health back to the extent where she could enjoy her life and be happy. I confess, I wanted the mother I never had, one who went to PTO meetings, volunteered in schools, took us to Girl Scouts, helped us with our homework, and read us bedtime stories. Like the traditional Indian woman, all my mother wanted was to fulfill her purpose as a wife and mother. When her family was happy, she was happy. When they weren't, she felt like a failure. She heard voices telling her she was a bad person and should die. When I was young, I would sometimes lay next to her and counter them, telling her she was a wonderful mother.

I chose to pursue osteopathic medicine and obtained a degree as a DO because I believed in the holistic approach, meaning treating the whole person. I always believed that there are many paths to healing. And for this reason, I had trouble accepting the black-and-white approach to medicine. When I took exams, I struggled with answering multiple-choice questions because I could come up with a possible scenario for each of the answers. To me, sometimes there is no one right answer. Human beings are complicated. The linear approach frustrated me. When I did my psychiatric rotation in my fourth year of medical school, I felt more at home.

Then my mother deteriorated, couldn't do much of anything for years, and died after being on a ventilator for six months. She had hypertensive heart disease and went into multi-organ failure. I never understood why. Why was her body on fire?

I completed a medical internship and a psychiatric residency with the final year as Chief Resident in 1994. I was well trained in psychotherapy and was on a track for psychoanalytic psychotherapy.

I didn't realize until many years later that I fervently approached every single patient as if they were my mother. In my way, I was trying to figure out what made her ill and what went wrong. I worked hard to get them well just like I wanted to get her well.

I approached each patient holistically, utilizing the biopsychosocial model proposed by George Engel and embraced by one of my mentors and past APA president, Paul Fink, M.D. I approached every patient by looking beyond the biology and the psychology – how one is also connecting and interacting socially, internally, and externally. I spent time trying to obtain an understanding of the psychological underpinnings of their symptoms and the dynamics of their relationships.

Over the years, I saw most of my patients in a community mental health center treating the chronic and persistent mentally ill, and I was the medical director at one such center for six years. I also worked in many different prison settings, from minimum to high security, treating substance use disorders, serious psychiatric disorders, and antisocial personality disorder. I worked on a geriatric psychiatry unit and in an outpatient setting for pregnant and postpartum women. I had a private practice doing psychotherapy and medication management. I've worked as a consultant/liaison psychiatrist on the medical floor in hospitals and in nursing homes. As a result, I gained years of experience running the entire gamut of psychiatric opportunities. These experiences laid the foundation for what I do now; bridge my conventional psychiatric training and experiences with functional medicine. Now I am at home.

It was a long journey to get here. Many years ago, I gathered a very thorough history of my patients including sleep, appetite, eating habits, and exercise. I addressed problems with drinking too much soda, coffee, or alcohol, smoking cigarettes and marijuana, and/or using other drugs. I taught deep breathing techniques, educated patients about sleep hygiene, the importance of making healthy choices in foods, cutting back on caffeine intake, and doing some exercise. Because some of my patients refused to see a primary care physician, I would often treat their medical issues, like hypothyroidism and hypertension. My initial evaluations were ninety minutes. I refused to do fifteen-minute med checks.

I ordered the appropriate labs and provided a detailed treatment plan – never just medications. I encouraged my patients to start a hobby or go out with friends, had discussions about spirituality, and addressed trauma issues and cognitive distortions. I made sure to follow up with their progress in these areas at most visits. Generally, I was satisfied that the symptoms I focused on remitted enough for patients to have some quality of life – to a point. After all, we believed that these were chronic and persistent mental illnesses. People regard me as a very good psychiatrist. I was even given the award of Exemplary Psychiatrist by NAMI Rhode Island in 2008 and became a Distinguished Fellow of the American Psychiatric Association.

I prescribed medications. Medications saved many lives and reduced immense suffering. I've had no choice at times – thankfully rare times – to use medications to sedate and restrain violent patients. I prided myself on reviewing the benefits and risks of medications that patients were already taking and took care in making sure they *all* were indicated and necessary, not just the psychiatric medications. I took care to make sure patients were not having side effects from the medications. I made sure that I did a med reconciliation on most visits. When taken long-term, medications can cause numerous and debilitating side effects.

Despite my diligence and efforts, it wasn't enough. I just couldn't figure out *why* some patients would reach a plateau and wouldn't improve further. Others were complete enigmas about whom other doctors were equally perplexed. I knew intuitively that I must be missing something. I knew it wasn't "in their heads," as some would say to me. Something was causing their suffering and I just couldn't put my finger on it. I wasn't satisfied. I was one of those people, and still am, who thinks most waking hours about my patients. They are puzzles that need to be solved. I knew that I needed to know more, and so the search for more training began.

In 2003, I began to have health issues. I sought care from my wonderful primary care provider. I couldn't function in a way that was my normal. I was exhausted. She initially told me "What do you expect?" I was obviously tired from raising three children and working a full-time job. That did not help me much, but what choice did I have? She drew bloodwork that gave me an answer. I had post-pregnancy Epstein Barr Virus and was in a thyroid storm, which caused a moderate depression. I was informed I had Hashimoto's thyroiditis. I was fortunate to have bloodwork to prove it, and my PCP then believed my distress. As an aside, I had evidence of having antibodies to my thyroid when I was in medical school in 1988 and was told to do nothing and to just monitor it. I know now that there are many things I could have done between 1988 to 2003 to prevent what happened in 2003. However, in 2003, I had a seemingly clear cause for depression, but given our training, there were no other alternatives known to us besides medication. I was stabilized on a high dose of levothyroxine and bupropion to address just those issues. This explained why I didn't lose the baby fat from my third child. I resigned myself to believe that this was permanent, and that I had no other choice but to accept it.

My husband is a professor of engineering at a local university. In 2010, he was up for sabbatical and we had a unique opportunity to go to France for two months. I said, "Well, you've never been to India in the thirty years we've been together and neither have the kids." I took leave from my job as a psychiatrist and medical director at the community mental health center, took the three kids out of school, and we lived in India for two months and then France for two months while my husband had an appointment at a French college. We homeschooled the kids and it was a fantastic once-in-a-lifetime trip. I highly recommend it. Talk about a living classroom! The kids had a blast and embraced it.

One day, in the last couple weeks of our trip, my boys had a tiff with each other in the apartment. Suddenly, one was gone. My son couldn't have gone far. I looked for him in the four rooms we had, but he was nowhere to be found. Then I saw the window open and there he was, standing on the ledge and ready to jump. I screamed, "What the heck are you doing? Are you crazy?" I was the mom, not the psychiatrist, at that moment. It didn't take much to get him back into the apartment. He was in tears and he was blubbering about missing his friends. I thought, *What the heck? He was fine minutes ago. What happened?* He was very depressed and anxious. There were other sudden changes that didn't make sense. He couldn't read anymore, and he had brain fog, and scattered thinking. This was so unlike the kid who, although he couldn't sit still, had good concentration and a photographic memory. He was in perfectly good health...or so I thought.

Of course, once we got home, I went down the usual path of trying to get him help. He saw a psychiatrist with a good reputation and initiated psychotherapy to address cognitive distortions connected to his anxiety. The medications abated his suicidal ideations and some of the depression. However, I couldn't figure out *why* this happened. Yeah, he had had some trouble making friends in the previous two years, but just before our trip to France, he had made some very good friends and he missed them while we were away. He was focused on them "forgetting about him" because the relationship was so new. But, it just didn't add up.

Around the same time, I was also exploring alternative therapies for my patients. I had a subset of patients who just weren't getting well. I knew I was missing something. Something was happening in their bodies that I just couldn't put my finger on. I had this same feeling with my son.

This search for alternative methods of treatment lead me to Visions Healthcare LLC in Dedham, Massachusetts in 2011. I asked Edward Levitan, M.D. to allow me to shadow him. I didn't know at the time that this honored request would completely change the trajectory of my life. I came to Dr. Levitan's office on Tuesday afternoons and was amazed at the types of patients he'd see, how he treated them, and how quickly they got better. I knew nothing about it. He practiced functional medicine; a model that helps us to identify the multiple-layered causes of symptoms that occur over a period of time and acknowledges the interconnected web of interactions that uncover the cause of the causes. People who practice functional medicine include conventional and integrative approaches, but they take it one step further.

I knew I had to bring my son to Dr. Levitan's office. My son was evaluated, and long story short, Dr. Levitan figured out *why* my son became depressed. He was found to have celiac disease, among other things. My son wasn't in the perfect health I had thought he was. I didn't realize that his lifelong problems of constipation and eczema weren't just a part of who he was or just *his* normal. Doctors prescribed laxatives and creams respectively but never explained or perhaps never were trained to understand why. I didn't know why either, but I certainly posed the question many times.

After treating my son with the functional medicine approach, which you will understand better in forthcoming chapters, it took up to a year for his depression to resolve. We were able to discontinue the three to four medications for depression, anxiety, sleep, and attention issues. It took two years for the double vision, which we determined was what prevented him from reading, to improve. This delayed his ability to get his driver's license. My son was unable to read or drive because his eye muscles were inflamed!

After working with Dr. Levitan, I came to understand the root causes of all my own health problems as well. I was no longer just stable on medication – my health improved dramatically, and I looked ten years younger. I felt great! I no longer needed to take four medications daily for environmental allergies. Over time, I was able to lower my dose of levothyroxine by half and tapered the dose of my antidepressant to nothing.

Once I saw the power of functional medicine, I couldn't turn back. I couldn't "unknow" this approach. It may not be lifesaving – like in an acute emergency – that's what conventional medicine does best. It is life-changing in other ways and saves your life in another sense, by improving the quality as well as quantity of years.

I asked to join Visions Healthcare in 2012. At the time, it was the largest functional medicine practice in the country. I loved working there and learned a great deal. I was a sponge and just couldn't stop soaking up every detail. I became addicted to information. I had to learn biochemistry, anatomy, and physiology again and actually apply these concepts in my assessment and treatment recommendations. I had always wondered why we learned these sciences in the first two years of medical school just to never use them again! I ultimately became a certified practitioner through the Institute for Functional Medicine. Unfortunately, Visions Healthcare had to close its doors in August 2015, so I partnered with Sally Davidson, ANP, and we opened a private practice called Functional Mind, LLC. We network with multiple-functional medical groups across the country and train medical students and nurse practitioners who are interested in learning this approach. We are always learning and always searching for new ways to improve people's health.

Because of these experiences over the last decade, I've concluded that there are certain circumstances when medications could be used emergently to stabilize someone, but then use functional medicine to figure out what went wrong, bring the body back into balance, and if possible reduce or discontinue medication (if and when warranted). I believe that this is an option that ought to be offered to patients.

Psychiatrists who are trained in a psychodynamic approach are well-positioned to becoming very good functional medicine practitioners as we think in *shades of gray*, rather than black and white. We can see layers of issues all at once and can predict how one event can affect and lead to a series of events. Even a simple infection that is treated with an antibiotic and resolved can be looked at differently by asking the question of *why?* Why did that person get an infection? Why does one person get sick all of the time and another person appear healthy despite smoking and drinking?

I sometimes fantasize about how my life would have been different had my mother been able to be the mother we needed, and she wanted to be. When I see women with mental and physical distress who have young children, I know firsthand that the children will be affected unless there is built-in support. I'm not minimizing the importance of the role of fathers. Mothers have traditionally been what bind family members to each other, the linchpin of society.

In retrospect, I know my mother would have had a significantly better quality of life as well, had we known about functional medicine before. She died the year before it was founded. I didn't believe my mother then when she said her improvement wasn't because of psychological reasons. Now I do believe her. From my son's history and my history, I can surmise what did make the difference in India. I know what the likely root causes were for her. Let's see if you can put the pieces together. I'll give you the big reveal on what I think they were at the back of the book. My hope is that my journey will serve others and her suffering would not have been in vain.

CHAPTER 3

How to Use This Book

*"Where attention goes, energy
flows and results show."*
– T. Harv Eker

I wrote this book specifically for the person who has fallen between the cracks, sitting in the void where there is seemingly no one to go to for help. This person is sick and tired, has gone to the doctor, has been told that their bloodwork is normal, has depression, and was presented with the option of taking a medication. I will show you how to figure out the major root causes of your own symptoms of distress by finding the puzzle pieces of your life that manifested them, and guide you through a different model of thinking about how to address these root causes (when you are stable). I might use the word "depression" interchangeably as a general term for mental distress and use the term "doctor" to include all practitioners who have prescribing privileges. By the end of the book, you will know what you need to do to effect a change in your symptoms that accompany and potentially cause mental distress. Depending on what you uncover and how much time and energy you invest, it could take as little as three months to see a difference in getting your mental and physical health back. As you're reading this book, there will be some things that you read and connect with right away because they're common sense to you. There might be other things that make sense initially, but you find you can't quite jive with the concept or concepts right away because it's a very different way of thinking.

It's like one of those famous optical illusions, The Young Woman, Old Woman Ambiguous Figure. You might see an old woman or a young woman based on your perceptions. They are both there, but it's a matter of how you look at it. My goal is not to discredit conventional medicine, but to offer another model. This other model takes an investment of time, energy, and money.

At the very least, I hope by reading Chapter 4, you can determine whether or not taking an antidepressant is the right decision for you right now. There is absolutely no shame in this, but I hope you have a full understanding of why you are taking them. Even if you choose to take medication, I hope that by reading the rest of the book, you will understand your options if they stop working, start having side effects, or if you decide you want to stop them at some point. It's best to be fully informed. Even if you choose to take medication, you can still determine the root causes of your symptoms while you work on feeling better and stronger with the medication.

Chapter 5 introduces you to that different model of thinking and way to approach this model. This doesn't mean you have to abandon the conventional model. They intersect or overlap nicely like yin and yang. They can dance with each – one leads and the other follows. Psychiatrists who are well-versed in psychotherapy and psychopharmacology know how to do that. When to wear one hat, or the other, or both. Functional medicine is yet another hat that I've learned to wear.

Chapter 6 will help you do a self-assessment and make a timeline of your history. *Be curious* about your own story like Sherlock Holmes and reflect on all of the things you've experienced. Take your time with it. Go back and add things when they occur to you. You might find that there have been many things going on in your body and mind for a while and that these things finally manifested themselves as mental distress. There is one assessment tool you will learn about called the Multiple Symptom Questionnaire. Make multiple copies of this tool and complete it on a monthly basis to mark your progress. I have all of my patients complete this tool as part of my Intake Packet as a baseline and then before every follow-up visit.

Chapter 7 will aid you in getting to know your body, how it literally functions mechanically, and getting those areas back online. You will approach your body in the same way you'd approach the engine of a car when checking the oil and the carburetor. It's a major layer, and much can change for you just from this one chapter!

Once you have completed the tasks in Chapter 7, you can choose to do any of the subsequent four chapters – Chapters 8 through 11 – in the order you wish, or you can do them concurrently. There is no right or wrong. There is testing that can be done at specific labs if you wish. I have included labs in the Appendix that you can ask your primary care provider to draw, but my experience is that most will not order them because they do not know why they are being ordered, how to interpret them, nor do they want to take responsibility for them. So, finding a functional medicine provider might be helpful. You can go to www.ifm.org and click on the link for Find A Practitioner. Don't let this issue prevent you from completing the other steps.

Chapter 12 provides steps to prevent recurrences. This is a very important chapter. Do *not* overlook it. By this point, many people feel better, drop out of treatment, and do not get to these steps. They get back into the rat race and eventually the symptoms return. Chapter 13 helps you re-evaluate the landscape and decide what areas of your life you need to protect at all costs to prevent a return of symptoms and what areas allow you more flexibility. Chapter 14 gives you tools to increase your awareness of your *being* as you look to the future, addresses your resistance, and helps you set your priorities. Chapter 15 invites you to celebrate and look forward to a better future.

The most important thing to keep in mind is to be patient with yourself and look at this process as a journey. It's not a silver bullet approach. Much of this process is educating yourself and changing habits.

I strongly recommend that you keep a journal. This recommendation is at the top of every initial treatment plan I give patients. I had a patient who worked with me in my practice and felt great but didn't write anything down. Six months later, she got stressed at her job, stopped doing all of the things that brought her body back into balance, and all of her symptoms returned and were even worse. The good news was that she knew that her results were achievable. Knowing that alone was "gold" to her. However, if she had written the steps down in her journal, it would have helped her to know which interventions were the most important to continue at all costs despite the stress, and which she could be more flexible about.

Please look at this as an adventure – a way of getting to know who you are and finding yourself in your health. This book is meant to get you thinking, to start your journey, and to give you hope. This book is not meant to be an exhaustive list of everything you need to address. It's very possible that you are further down on your journey and are experiencing something I don't even mention. Please don't let that invalidate your experience. There is much that I explore with my patients that I haven't even mentioned.

If you do this work, it can take as little as three months to feel great. The average person in my practice, if they stay on course, takes six to twelve months. If it takes longer, then there are other factors involved that require further investigation with someone who has experience in figuring these sorts of things out. The types of issues that take longer for the body to heal include chronic unremitting stress, childhood trauma that still plays an active role in your current life, self-hatred, acute illnesses, traumatic brain injuries, Lyme disease, small intestine bacterial overgrowth, multiple chemical sensitivities, mast cell activation syndrome, postural orthostatic tachycardia syndrome, Ehlers Danlos syndrome, autoimmune illnesses, chronic fatigue syndrome, chronic pain, autism, mold exposure, and toxicity. Some people have three to four of these issues all at the same time. Doing these steps certainly helps to improve these conditions but it can take several years to resolve these issues.

CHAPTER 4

Why You Were Given a Prescription

want you to know that you aren't going crazy and you aren't alone. Thousands of people have experienced what you are experiencing. I want to acknowledge and validate your feelings of confusion, helplessness, and frustration. These feelings alone can cause a person to feel distressed mentally. Instead of the word "depressed" to describe their emotions, I prefer that people find words that express their emotions more precisely.

Here is a list of 100 words to choose: abandoned, achy, afraid, agitated, agony, alone, anguish, antisocial, anxious, breakdown, brittle, broken, catatonic, consumed, crisis, crushed, crying, defeated, defensive, dejected, demoralized, desolate, despair, desperate, despondent, devastated, discontented, disheartened, dismal, distractible, distraught, distressed, doomed, dreadful, dreary, edgy, emotional, empty, excluded, exhausted, exposed, fatalistic, forlorn, fragile, freaking, gloomy, grouchy, helpless, hopeless, hurt, inadequate, inconsolable, injured, insecure, irrational, irritable, isolated, lonely, lousy, low, melancholy, miserable, moody, morbid, needy, nervous, nightmarish, oppressed, overwhelmed, pain, paranoid, pessimistic, reckless, rejected, resigned, sad, self-conscious, self-disgust, shattered, stagnant, sobbing, sorrowful, suffering, suicidal, tearful, touchy, trapped, uneasy, unhappy, unhinged, unpredictable, upset, vulnerable, wailing, weak, weepy, withdrawn, woeful, wounded, wretched, zonked.

As you read them, you've probably had some of these feelings at some time in your life. They describe a normal human experience. Poets write about these feelings. These are normal feelings; dare I say, it's even normal to occasionally have *fleeting* suicidal thoughts. All of these emotions need to be put in context. Don't get me wrong, I am not suggesting that you ignore these thoughts. I have had patients who use only one word to describe their emotions and that one word is depressed. I have to show them the list of words to really get them to describe what they are truly feeling; that's half the battle. Sometimes just telling someone it's normal to feel this way causes *huge* relief. This takes time to sort out.

Let me help you to understand where the disconnect is between you and your doctor. You've got a prescription, but you don't know *why* your doctor gave it to you – or she said you were depressed but you don't believe it. According to *The Annals of Family Medicine*, doctors spend an average of seventeen minutes with each patient to discern the problem. They use a decision tree, a tree-like model of "if this, then that," to arrive at a diagnosis so they know how to match a "pill to the ill." They might also do the PHQ-9, which is a questionnaire to quickly see if you meet the criteria for clinical depression. If you score high enough, it gives the doctor the confidence to prescribe medication. Why? Because there are studies that tell them that there is validity to this questionnaire and it's an efficient method to provide a quick solution. It's evidence-based, meaning that there are studies that give it validation and it meets the standard of care. They might add some supportive advice, like "take time for yourself" or "you're too hard on yourself" or "you need to get more sleep" because the belief is that medication will do the rest and there is little *time* to do anything else. Doing blood work to rule out medical causes of depression is the standard of care.

The medical model identifies a cluster of symptoms to provide a diagnosis, that helps to quickly decide how to treat a problem. This works very well for acute or emergency issues and is useful for quick decisions about which medications would be most appropriate. Psychiatrists do a more thorough evaluation, but the outcome is generally the same. A severe clinical depression is a very serious condition that can potentially end up in suicide, or harm to others for that matter. Safety always comes first. Therefore, identifying it and acting quickly to be sure that a person is treated appropriately and safely is paramount. Psychiatrists tend not to see people like Katie.

Nowadays, however, antidepressants are being used for many conditions beyond depression. For the purposes of this book, I will explain how I decide if someone must take medication for a clinical depression.

One type of depression is more formally known in the DSM-5 as major depression. It typically has at least five of the following symptoms *all day, every day* for at least two weeks, and at least one of the symptoms should be either depressed mood or loss of interest or pleasure.

- Distinctly depressed/irritable mood or *marked* loss of interest/pleasure
- Decreased or increased weight or appetite
- Appearing slowed or agitated

- Fatigue or loss of energy
- Feeling worthless or guilty
- Poor concentration or indecisiveness
- Thoughts of death, suicide attempts, or plans

It's assumed that medical causes or substance use have been ruled out prior to a depression diagnosis but many times, antidepressants are prescribed despite this. For example, many doctors acknowledge the effects of alcohol on mood acutely and chronically. Technically, they ought not be giving a diagnosis of a depressive disorder until alcohol and drugs are removed.

I strongly recommend offering antidepressant medications when someone has been feeling so depressed that they can't function, can't get out of bed, are having daily crying spells, are actively or chronically suicidal, making poor decisions, and/or behaving in a way they cannot control, which might threaten failure in school, destruction of relationship or a loss of their job. However, emotional distress is quite subjective and if a patient felt strongly that they wanted medication and from my perspective met the appropriate criteria, I would prescribe it with the proper informed consent, also offering alternatives. Medication can take as little as two weeks to provide an effect, but on average, it takes four to six weeks. Sometimes, it takes eight weeks, but after eight weeks at a therapeutic dose without an effect, it's considered a failed trial. Any benefit prior to two weeks might be considered the placebo effect, but even that is controversial.

In the meantime, what I do differently from other psychiatrists, if a patient is able and willing, is to dive deep searching for root causes so that patients might avoid or be able to stop relying on medication. Therefore, if you meet those criteria, the benefits do outweigh the risks, especially if you have a family history of depression. It sometimes helps to give a person a diagnosis because they can then search for other solutions in the meantime. Other treatment options, depending on the severity, include electroconvulsive therapy and transcranial magnetic stimulation. However, providing a diagnosis can also hurt a person if they have family members with depression; they assume they will follow the same chronic path and believe there is no solution. This outlook decreases their chances of looking for alternatives. I believe having a diagnosis is a starting point to understand and convey what you are experiencing, but it shouldn't define you, label you, or give you a feeling that you will always have a diagnosis for the rest of your life. Sometimes, it is not helpful to give a person a diagnosis if it's going to interfere with the healing process. My experience is that if you can find the root causes of the symptoms and rectify the problem, the emotional distress will go away. The decision to take an antidepressant is generally determined by how much distress you're experiencing, how difficult it is for you to function, and the risk of suicide. If taking medication in the meantime helps to relieve symptoms, and it's well tolerated without side effects, that's great. Take the medication, but do what you can to figure out *why!*

Years ago, in my early training, we as psychiatrists spent significant time with our patients to understand what they were experiencing and why. We had some medications, tricyclic and monoamine oxidase inhibitors, that we could use, but we weren't reliant on them for milder forms of depression because of severe side effects. The benefits didn't outweigh the risks. Instead, we did psychotherapy. Then a new class of medications starting with Prozac hit the market in 1987. A lot of people who were battling depression at the time were in weekly psychotherapy and possibly taking the older antide-pressants that were, because of their dangerous side effects, typically prescribed only by psychiatrists. The relative safety of the newer class of antidepressants changed everything. Some people who were in long-term psychotherapy got better with the newer class of antidepressants and subsequently dropped out of psychotherapy. The side effect profile reduced the risk of death from overdose as compared to the older medications. They were miracle pills...but there were few to no studies about how or why they worked, long-term effectiveness, or long-term side effects, even now. The sessions became shorter and shorter. It didn't matter what label of depression you had; you still were prescribed an SSRI. Because of a shortage of psychiatrists and the safety profile, family doctors began to prescribe SSRIs. This was followed in 1997 with the first advertisements on TV for medications, persuading the public to talk to their doctors to prescribe them. This combination of circumstances triggered an explosion of prescriptions for antidepressants. Your appointment time was no longer about the relationship with your doctor, which in itself has great healing power. The act of listening, connecting, acknowledging, and validation alone can be very healing. The sense of being heard and reassured is healing. This is a huge loss in our system because of the lack of time. As a result, some people leave their doctor's office feeling worse than when they arrived and others go to the doctor just to acquire a prescription. Slowly over the years, who you were as a person, what you experienced, and what you wanted didn't matter. It could all be solved with a pill. It was just a matter of picking the right pill, the right dose or the right combination of pills. Each session with the doctor was a tweak here and a tweak there. If one SSRI didn't work, then another one was tried. Then the

Serotonin and Norepinephrine Reuptake Inhibitors (SNRIs), a class of antidepressants, were launched. They were used as a second line of treatment if SSRIs didn't work. And if they didn't work, other medications were used as adjuvants to boost the antidepressant. And if they didn't work, they called the depression, "treatment resistant," which some people interpret as "this is your fault." And then you're at a dead end.

I like to use a lightbulb analogy to explain. If you were sitting on the couch reading a book and the lightbulb went out, you would assume that the lightbulb died. After changing the lightbulb, if the new one didn't come on, you might think that one was dead, too. Would you keep doing the same thing after the third lightbulb? When it comes to antidepressants, your average doctor would just keep changing the antidepressant or they'd refer you to a psychiatrist and then *they* would keep changing the antidepressant.

So, think about what you'd do if after the third lightbulb didn't work. Barring the possibility that the whole package of lightbulbs was damaged, you might look to see if the cord was plugged in, if the wall switch was switched on, check other electrical items in the house were working, and even look outside to see if others' houses were affected. Common sense, right?

This type of thinking is less prevalent now in conventional medicine. Sherlock Holmes of conventional medicine is virtually extinct. When doctors do venture into this type of thinking, it's on their own time and they don't get paid. The health insurance industry responded on some level to pay for time, but in return required an enormous amount of paperwork to back it up, and the increase in reimbursement was miniscule in comparison. There was a time (and this still is an issue with some insurances) when they stated that statistically one only needed six sessions of psychotherapy. A study had shown that the *average* person went to six sessions of psychotherapy and dropped out. They thus presumed that six sessions were all that they needed.

What has changed over the last fifty years is our environment. Our medical system rarely addresses this or even acknowledges it. We have been inundated by processed foods since the advent of Betty Crocker's cake mix, margarine, and processed and artificial sugars. We have been exposed to the production of thousands of new chemicals every year in our air, soil, products, and food supply. Finally, our society has become driven by our culture to make more money at the expense of our health with long hours of work, no lunch breaks, and little vacation time. The medical system is aware of the impact of the opiate crisis, of antibiotics causing antibiotic resistance, and of polypharmacy (prescribing too many medications). Health Research Funding reported in June 2017 that polypharmacy accounts for almost thirty percent of all hospital admissions and is the fifth leading cause of death in the US. Doctors don't know how to fix it other than prescribing fewer opiates, antibiotics, or medications in general. All of these factors can ultimately impact you and result in mental distress.

Are you familiar with the bell curve? It is called this for its distinctive shape resembling the Liberty Bell. It suggests that most cases fall in the mid-range with relatively few at the margins. Most people fall under the bell curve and all studies are based on how the *average* person responds to the medication. And by the way, in studies with regard to effectiveness, a fifty percent response to antidepressant medication is considered a success.

What happens to the bottom half? You get lost in the background and continue to search and suffer. It's this person who searches for answers and finds functional medicine. It's a person like Katie who is well enough that she doesn't *require* the antidepressant and wants to get right down to finding the root causes.

At its basic level, mental distress or depression is a symptom telling you something is wrong. It's a red flag saying, "Pay attention." Pure and simple. Something is wrong in your mind, your body, your environment, and/or your soul. It can be a normal reaction to an event in your life but if the timing of that event collides with another stressful event, the reaction may not be within the range of normal.

There are numerous causes of depression and I've listed many of them from a bio-psychosocial perspective. Again, this is not an exhaustive list; it's just to get you thinking.

- Biological:

  o Conventional medications: most commonly benzodiazepines like Xanax, barbiturates, opiates, anti-epileptic drugs, beta blockers, corticosteroids, anti-virals like interferon alpha and beta, isotretinoin (used to treat acne), varenicline (used to quit smoking), and even the antidepressant bupropion.

  o The most well-known medical conditions investigated by your doctor are as follows: hypothyroidism, hyperparathyroidism, B12 deficiency, and folate deficiency. More obvious conditions obtained by history are stroke, seizures, or traumatic brain injury. Less common are Cushing's syndrome, Addison's disease, Huntington's disease, Wilson's disease, multiple sclerosis, Parkinson's disease, HIV, West Nile virus, Creutzfeldt-Jakob disease, Lyme disease, neurosyphilis, Hepatitis C, paraneoplastic syndromes, and pancreatic cancer. These are major diseases that can cause *severe* depression and can be ruled out.

This might explain why the patient is told that they've ruled out a medical cause.

- Psychosocial:
  - Existential crisis, mid-life crisis
  - Period of regression before personal growth
  - Internal conflicts and perception of self and others
  - Chronic automatic negative thoughts
  - Lack of direction and purpose
  - Lack or problem with sense of self including sexuality or self-hatred
  - Lack or problem with attachment, connection and community
  - Lack of trust or betrayal
  - Sadness or grief from loss or death
  - Chronic feelings of guilt, fear, shame or anger
  - Reactions to feelings and reactions to reactions
  - Current or past physical, sexual, or emotional abuse
  - Conflict in relationship – ranging from passive to aggressive. Feeling "unseen," invalidated, or "gaslighting" can be as damaging as shouting matches
  - Major events like moving, losing a job or income, getting divorced, or retiring. Even joyful events such as starting a new job, graduating, getting married, or having a baby
  - Social isolation or lack of acceptance by society
  - Serious illnesses – direct contribution of and/or

difficulty managing the illness

- o Substance abuse – drugs or alcohol temporarily may cause you feel better, but ultimately can cause depression

What's missing is the functional medicine perspective, added below in no particular order.

- Hypoglycemia and other blood sugar dysregulations
- Inflammation and immune system dysregulation
- Energy regulation and mitochondrial dysfunction (how you make energy)
- Biotransformation and elimination (how you detox)
- Nutritional deficiencies and digestive difficulties
- Food sensitivities, food and environmental allergies, and poor diet (GMO foods, processed food, and sugar)
- Assessment of the microbiome
- Irritable bowel syndrome, chronic bacterial, viral, parasitic or fungal infection, small intestine bacterial overgrowth or any gut infection
- Environmental toxins (occupational, household cleansers, pesticides, and cosmetics)
- Hormonal and neurotransmitter dysregulation and communication between systems
- Impact of stress on the body
- Transportation highway of the cardiovascular system and lymphatic system
- Structural integrity from subcellular membranes to mucosal structure
- Genetic variability that makes one more susceptible to not being able to utilize nutrients that are synthetic
- Genetic variability that causes some people to have

> higher requirements of specific nutrients (for example, zinc or Vitamin B6)

Just listing them here doesn't do it justice because it doesn't demonstrate the dynamics of the system at play and the interplay between them over time. I will touch on this list in more detail in subsequent chapters.

As you might surmise, depression has many causes. If you look at the lists above, there are likely multiple things you could circle that affect you currently or have in the past. It's important to note what you had in the past because it may have just gone below the surface of your awareness or your body was able to put that in check, but other symptoms came to the surface. Knowing what conditions you had in the past helps to put the pieces of the puzzle together. Make your own list in your journal. Put a C for "current" and a P for "past" next to the factors listed above, and if you have a factor in the past and still have it currently, put both there.

We talked about the fact that depression is a symptom in the body telling you something is wrong, and that there are multiple ways that depression can show up in your life. So, why doesn't your doctor look at all of these factors and come up with a plan?

Perhaps I can illustrate an example. Sometimes when a patient sees a doctor, they might get some blood work for their annual exam. The doctor might note the blood sugar slightly elevated and ask about family history. They might mention diet and exercise, but not *how* to implement a diet and exercise or which foods and which exercises are best for this (because they don't have the time nor the training). If they are good, they might refer you to a nutritionist, but then say, "We'll watch it." Next year, the blood sugar is slightly more elevated, and they might say the same thing. The following year, your blood sugar is so elevated that your Hemoglobin A1C is elevated. Then they will give you a diagnosis that makes it medically necessary for treatment and then they can match a pill, an oral hypoglycemic, or insulin if it's bad enough. By this point, it's usually too late to save your pancreas and reverse the process. What fails to get translated in this process is that if you catch elevated blood sugars early enough, you absolutely can reverse the condition.

Why didn't the doctor investigate *why* the blood sugars are elevated? Why didn't the doctor educate the patient in detail of the importance of what needs to be done and why? Because insurance only pays for things that are medically necessary and doctors aren't typically trained in nutrition and exercise; they aren't adequately trained in prevention.

Many people don't understand the role of the medical system. They do understand how auto insurance and home insurance work. People know that they can't use these insurances to paint their house, seal their driveway, or fix the toilet. Think about what would happen if you did absolutely nothing for your car except put gasoline in it. Believe me, there are people who do that! How long would it last? Eventually it would rust, work inefficiently, start smoking, the brakes would fail, and the tires would get bald.

Most people don't realize that their medical insurance, the way it was originally intended, is not meant to pay for the upkeep of the body, mind, and soul. The explosion of people with chronic symptoms like Katie's, which are now labeled depression, are different from the people with depression from the 1950s. They don't realize that most people with this type of depression have not been doing the upkeep in terms of diet, sleep, exercise, stress, and toxin exposure.

You see, most of your chronic symptoms, depression being one of them, are due to your diet and lifestyle. It's only when depression gets so bad that it becomes debilitating that the problem gets addressed. It used to be that medications were only offered once it reached a certain threshold, but that threshold has been lowered again and again over the years. The antidepressant medications are also used to treat other conditions like panic disorder, OCD, and other anxiety disorders, among other things.

The void is where people fall who aren't sick enough to get the attention of psychiatrists but are feeling something is wrong with them. This feeling might be described as "being off," "out of it," or "apathetic." These aren't psychiatric diagnoses. When someone presents with these quoted descriptions chronically with enough physical symptoms on repeated visits to a doctor, the doctor might give a prescription for an antidepressant because they don't have anything else to offer and not enough time to figure it out. Sometimes, some doctors give an antidepressant for what we call a "wastebasket" diagnosis, because they just don't know what else to offer.

This is not an appropriate reason to give an antidepressant. It is appropriate to give an antidepressant when it is indicated for a documented psychiatric condition that interferes in personal, social, and occupational functioning after all medical causes are ruled out, and when the benefits outweigh the risks. There is nothing wrong with a trial of an antidepressant, and if it helps you, great! Medications work some of the time for some people. Some people can't take medication because it causes side effects. Some people just don't want an antidepressant.

In the functional medicine approach, one looks for the root cause or causes of the problem and brings the body back into balance by finding and addressing each root cause, so you won't have to take medication at all or long-term. Another bonus is that you learn what factors mitigated those symptoms, and you know what to do for the rest of your life.

Looking at the timeline of how the diagnosis and treatment of depression evolved is a demonstration of what influenced thinking in our society. It's a macroscopic example of what happens in the body. My hope is that you were able to appreciate the complexities of depression. Depression at its basic level is a symptom. It is on a continuum of severity like the volume knob on the radio. Severity can lead to a clinical diagnosis. The goal of this chapter was to inform you about why a doctor might think you were depressed and provide a prescription, to determine if this action was indeed appropriate for you, to determine what's changed over the years that might be contributing to your mental and physical distress, and to give you hope that there is an alternative approach.

CHAPTER 5

A Paradigm Shift

There was a time when, if you needed to get from one place to another and didn't have a friend to help you out, you likely would have called a taxi. The classic Yellow Cab driver was highly regulated and part of a larger organization. They didn't work independently, and it was very difficult to become a cab driver because of the cost of a medallion. There are areas in the country where taxis didn't even exist. They tended to be in major cities. So, the idea that someone in your town can be called up to transport you somewhere in minutes was a new frontier.

Uber was officially launched in 2011. This rocked the taxi establishment, as there was clearly a demand. Similarly, functional medicine is rocking the current medical establishment because of strong demand. This *Uberization* of medicine began with on-demand access to doctors via apps and online technology, but it has evolved into the *quality* of care as well.

I hope you see that depression is a symptom – a way the body tells you there is a problem. It could be something that has been there on a low level for years and fluctuates over time, or it could be a new symptom that has compounded on top of other issues that you've just been powering through. When most people get the flu, they get depressed. That's a normal process of the flu in the body. The influenza virus is at war with your immune system.

Inflammation can cause many different symptoms. Many times, causes are linked to each other by how much inflammation they produce in the body. It can just make you feel "blah!" You will learn more about this in Chapter 7. We might have to remove some things that are inflaming the body, add some things that the body needs to work efficiently, support the immune system to work efficiently with the microbiome and optimally, repair some areas of the body on a cellular level.

Although you might have things going on that you can point to that are legitimately causing you to feel down or depressed, like a break-up or someone close to you passing away, having inflammation in the body is a layer that makes those losses feel even worse. Think about handling a difficult problem and then think about handling that same problem while you have a headache. Doesn't it feel harder to do? The chronicity and severity of symptoms tells you how long it's been there and the approximate number of layers.

Sid Baker, M.D., an early contributor to functional medicine, talked about the TACKS rule. If you're sitting on a tack, it takes a lot of aspirin to make it feel good! If you're sitting on two tacks, removing one does not make it feel fifty percent better. You need to remove all the tacks to feel better. Some people live with symptoms they think are normal, and over the years, they may accumulate these tacks until their body feels like it's struggling. Everyone has a different level of tolerance or a different "pain" point as some people call it. It's the point in your life when you might say "enough is enough", and this becomes a watershed moment.

As you live your life, the challenges you contend with daily accumulate over time. The rain barrel effect has to do with how a rain barrel is used. A rain barrel is usually hooked up to the drain of your house. It collects rainwater, and once it is full, one might water the garden with the water. After a particular storm that had significant rainfall, that rain barrel might overflow. Normally, you'd want to watch the level of the water in the barrel and use that water up before the next storm. By way of analogy, you do want to do the same in life. If you have had a rough "storm" in your life, you will want to drain that barrel before it overflows. Sometimes, people forget that they had a rain barrel and don't tend to it. When it overflows, it might destroy the land around it through flooding. Managing the rain barrel is like managing life. Even if you're good at it, you might have two or three big stressors come together that create your "perfect storm" that causes your immune system to crash. For me, it was being postpartum, then EBV, and autoimmune thyroiditis, all on top of the stress of a new job. For my son, he had severe constipation, severe eczema, and physical restlessness for years, and the storm occurred when he hit puberty.

Just because you aren't feeling something doesn't mean it's not happening. My friend David said to me, "I'm fine except I have [environmental] allergies. I didn't have allergies last year." There is an assumption that if a person is having a problem that it is *always* caused by something outside of themselves. David assumed that if he is having sniffles that it is definitely due to something environmental. However, it could be a breach in his gut lining, hypochlorhydria, or sensitivities to food with cross-reactivity to the environment. It is possible that he had a sensitivity to trees all along, but his immune system did a really good job hiding it from him. Then it came to his attention because his immune system was stressed and now it is unable to do as good a job. What caused the stress that overloaded his system? Not sleeping as well due to stresses of his job, his daughter getting married, and caring for his elderly parents.

Conventional medicine tends to address things downstream and functional medicine tends to address things upstream. As an example, think about a river going down the side of a mountain. People are camping all along the river. There might be a great water hole in a cove where people like to bathe and enjoy the water. If people upstream started to dump food and garbage in the water, it would affect the people downstream. It would be disgusting to have things floating by and accumulating on the rocks. It would smell. The park could hire a crew to clean it up daily or hourly even, charge people money to use the park, and say, "That's the way it is. That's life, you gotta live with it." Or they could go upstream and tell those people that they have to stop dumping garbage into the river or they'd be fined. There is no right or wrong. Either option is fine, but one option is prevention and the other option is to live with it or fix the damage when it happens.

Another thing most people don't realize is that the body can heal itself. Conventional medicine tells us that the body makes mistakes and can't be fixed. That once you have a diagnosis, you can't turn back. That's true if you've let things go beyond a point and not addressed them. Do you remember my example of elevated blood sugars? If you cleared something upstream, removed the barriers, and provided the nutrients that the body needs to function efficiently, it wouldn't tax the system to the point of burning out the pancreas forcing you to take medications. Yes, there is a small percentage of people who have genetic problems that cause them to need insulin. The majority of people would not need these medications if they searched for the cause upstream.

When we cut ourselves, the bleeding stops within minutes. Within days, there is a scab. That, believe it or not, is an example of what our body shows it can do. Our body is constantly working to manage the barrier between our cells and the outside environment. Every inch of our bodies is covered with the microbiome, an integral part of the immune system that keeps everything from attacking or invading us. We need to consider that the body's reaction to a breach is the immune system functioning appropriately. We wouldn't live long if we didn't have our immune system. The immune system has two roles: defense and repair.

Our immune system functions optimally when the host is happy, provided the raw materials to function efficiently, allowed to rest, fills its reserves, and the barriers to healing are lifted.

Conventional doctors are focused on diagnosis – *what* is it? That is just a name for it. Functional medicine doctors look for the underlying cause and focus on the *why*. One diagnosis can have multiple root or underlying causes, and multiple conventional diagnoses can have one root cause.

A person who I recently evaluated who had a chief complaint with depression had all of the following root causes and they each needed to be addressed:

- A diet high in processed carbohydrates that caused her to have episodes of hypoglycemia
- Copper toxicity and copper/zinc imbalance. To rule out the severity of the copper toxicity, we did a kryptopyrrole test to rule out pyroluria. Genetically, this will mean taking high doses of zinc and Vitamin B6 lifelong.

- A Candida infection
- High stress related to her job, negative thoughts, and distorted self-perception. Due to the high stress, she likely was not digesting her food. We tested for hypochlorhydria to determine that.

Conventional doctors might not examine any of those four root causes except perhaps the hypoglycemia – and that typically is discovered only after taking a detailed history.

It's not one-size-fits-all, but you get one pill to fix a diagnosis. The body is enormously complicated, and the reasons why it is out of balance are as varied and unique on the inside as it is on the outside. Your house, car, decorations, clothes, body, ideas, and emotions are all unique. How can we think that a pill can fix everyone? Because of this mindset, people are on a laundry list of pills to target specific ills rather than looking upstream for the cause. As per my analogy, that would be like having a plan of action for each of the types of items dumped in the river and the problem they caused.

Aside from taking vitals, conventional doctors tend to minimize the importance of looking at the natural rhythms in the body and minimize dynamics and physiological changes in the body on a *chronic* basis. Conventional medicine does a spectacular job of responding to extreme changes but less well at responding to mild or moderate changes that might be indicative of a chronic problem that may be agitating the immune system. There are processes in the body that are always agitating the immune system. There is a dynamic interplay between hormones, neurotransmitters, circulation, digestion, and the microbiome that occur beautifully like an orchestra. A functional medicine doctor is concerned with how the orchestra is playing and that it is playing music beautifully.

If an instrument is off rhythm or key, the maestro finds it and corrects it.

What is normal? According to the WHO (World Health Organization), mental health is "… a state of well-being in which the individual realizes his or her own abilities, can cope with the normal stresses of life, can work productively and fruitfully, and is able to make a contribution to his or her community."

In the field of psychology, we have numerous models for how to approach an understanding of the mind – biological, behavioral, cognitive, humanistic, psychodynamic, sociocultural, evolutionary, and biopsychosocial. There is no one right model. They might overlap or build upon each other or even contradict. Most psychologists and psychiatrists accept them and might even switch from one model to another if something doesn't quite feel right. It's because we have multiple models to work with that we are able to understand and create effective solutions. Multiple models reflect the complexity and richness of the human mind.

Allopathic medicine, or modern medicine, is the prevailing model of thinking that has successfully stifled alternative models of care, such as osteopathy, homeopathy, and Ayurveda. Although integrative medicine has taken a foothold in some areas, it hasn't actually changed the model of thinking.

Over the years, functional medicine has been demanded by people frustrated by a failing medical system with a model that has many limitations. Although there is an important place for medications and surgery, when used in emergencies and acute situations, I see the field of functional medicine becoming the yin to the yang of conventional medicine someday, and taking its place in the forefront for addressing chronic conditions. As I've mentioned, functional medicine requires an investment of time and energy. It's not a quick fix, but it does allow you to have long-lasting results that improve multiple areas of the body and mind with the symptom(s) of depression likely being just one of them. It also takes believing in yourself and believing you are worth it. This takes work on your part. This is the paradigm shift people are demanding and is exemplified by recent changes on the horizon. At a top tech May 2019 conference in Silicon Valley, functional medicine was deemed the number one trend to watch. I call it the *Uberization* of medicine.

CHAPTER 6

Investigative Tools

Let's see what *is* going on in your body without having to label it. Remember, labels or diagnoses are for matching a pill to an ill, insurance coding, and doing research.

I find it helpful to put things on a timeline. We are going to list everything that has ever happened to you, large or small, to see what all the layers of issues that you have from even before you were born. I did this with my patients even before I started functional medicine. Details of a person's life allowed me to paint a picture of their issues in my mind. Psychiatric residents are trained to do this and it's especially helpful for doing psychotherapy, although we would write it in a narrative form to lay out a story of the person. Once I started doing functional medicine, I started to add in the information that we gather as functional medicine doctors and put it on a timeline. So, let's get started!

Get a large piece of paper. Place the paper with the long side horizontally. Then, draw a line horizontally in the center leaving an inch to the left. It doesn't have to be exact. Put zero on the left side of the line and put your age at the end of the line to the right. Then draw a vertical line for every decade that you were alive. So, if you are fifty-six, then you will have five lines for each decade and then leave space for the last six years.

In the top left corner, jot down what runs in your family – genetic or acquired.

What part of the world did your family originate from?

Are there any hereditary problems that you know about? For example, thalassemia or hemochromatosis?

Was there abuse in the family that was passed down? Alcoholism? Smoking? Anything else you can think of that was already there before you came into the world.

Now, no judgment allowed. Just the facts. Put on your Sherlock Holmes hat.

Go through the following list and jot it down on the timeline if you had it or have it. Draw a vertical line in the approximate location and put the item at the top and the date or age or both at the bottom.

If you don't know or need to ask your parents, then put a "?" or "Ask ____" next to it.

Before the number zero is where you put any information you had about your mother's pregnancy. How was the pregnancy in general? Did she have morning sickness? Was she on medication? Was she stressed? How was the delivery? Were there any complications?

Then, starting at zero, write down your birthday. Were you delivered naturally or via C-section? Were you breastfed or bottle-fed? For how long? Did you have any complications?

How were the first two years of life? Did you have colic? Did you have any problems tolerating formulas? Foods? Did you have any constipation?

If you had problems tolerating certain foods, did they go away? If so, at what age?

Did you have any ear infections? Throat infections? Sinus infections? Bronchitis? UTIs? Skin infections? Add any type of infection to the timeline. Have you had any viruses like mono due to EBV, Lyme's disease, or yeast/fungal infections (vaginal, toes, groin or jock itch)? Have you had mold exposure? If you've had yeast infections, complete the Candida Questionnaire in Chapter 8.

Do you have chronic sinus issues or a runny nose?

Did you receive any antibiotics during your life? Especially list if there have been repeated trials of antibiotics or long periods of taking antibiotics (e.g., doxycycline) for acne or prevention of malaria while traveling in a foreign country.

Did you fall and hit your head as a child? Need stitches? Did you play sports that caused you to have repeated hits to the head? Soccer? Football? Any motor vehicle accidents? Any concussions? Seizures?

Did you have any stomachaches, abdominal pain? Problems with constipation? Diarrhea?

Did you have eczema or acne?

Were there periods of issues with attention or restlessness?

If you are female, when did your menses begin? Was it heavy? Cramping? Painful?

If you are male, during puberty, did you have anything happen emotionally or physically during that time?

Did you have any surgeries? Add what the surgeries were on the timeline. If you have had a gastric bypass or colon resection, or your gallbladder removed, put those in red. Did you have your wisdom teeth removed? Have you had any mercury fillings, root canals, or crowns/implants inserted? Have you had anything put into your body, e.g., breast implants, titanium rods, or IUDs?

Across the top, add a squiggly line for periods of stress that affected you negatively. There could be breaks in the line where there was little to no stress. A stressful time could be growing up in a chaotic stressful household, middle school bullying, difficulty learning, high school academics, applying for colleges, college academics, exam periods, toxic work environment, unhealthy marriages, divorces, raising children without support, or working two jobs. Caretaking for a sick person or elderly person? Losses and their impacts – people, finances, etcetera. I use a life stress questionnaire in my practice to get an idea of the level of stress a person is experiencing. Here is a link to The Holmes-Rahe Stress Inventory to see how stress impacts your life: https://www.stress.org/holmes-rahe-stress-inventory-pdf.

To score this questionnaire, the following chart will give you some idea of how to informally score yourself.

300+	Indicates a high susceptibility to a health-related illness
150–299	Indicates a moderate susceptibility to a health-related illness
Less than 150	Indicates a low susceptibility to a health-related illness.

The higher your life change score, the harder you have to work to get yourself back into a state of good health. Stress reduction will be a major part of your plan to regain your health.

Also add unhealthy periods of coping with trauma and its impact. If you've experienced trauma, do the ACE score and Resilience score and learn about Adverse Childhood Events at this link: https://www.acesconnection.com/blog/got-your-ace-resilience-scores. This web resource provides free tools to get your ACE score and Resilience score.

Smoking – even if it's one cigarette a day – can trigger a chronic inflammatory agitation of your system. Drinking alcohol and using drugs, even used at low levels chronically can cause inflammation and impact your mood. (If you drink more than a couple of glasses of alcohol a week, write it down. It doesn't mean you are an alcoholic, but it is considered a toxin and it causes vitamin deficiencies and inflammation to the gut lining.) Also, even though marijuana is legal in some states, and has been touted to have health benefits, it can be a toxin for some people. It can cause paranoia and trigger psychotic episodes in susceptible people. Again, no judgment. We want to figure out how things impact your body. Think about it this way; if you started very gently scratching the top of one hand with the other and didn't stop, what would happen? It would become irritated, inflamed, maybe break your skin, and at some point, bleed. It would not heal until you stop scratching. The only way to start the healing process is to stop the irritation, no matter how small.

Have you had any environmental allergies and/or food allergies, sensitivities, or intolerances? Write down when you became aware of them. The food sensitivities that you had in the first two years of life are important clues even if you "grew out of them."

Have you been diagnosed with any issues like migraines, hypertension, high cholesterol, thyroid problems, or an auto-immune problem? Put it on the start date and a line for how long it has been a problem.

Have you had any weight gain or weight loss? Any difficulty in your ability to change your weight despite making concerted efforts when in the past, you've had no problem? Coping with food or restriction of food?

What about other hormonal changes like menopause or

andropause? When did they occur?

Last but not least, when did you have periods of anxiety, panic attacks, dysphoria, mood swings, or even psychosis?

This is not an exhaustive list, but I've listed the most important items to gather. I typically give my patients a thirty-nine-page intake to gather this type of information and I put the information they provide on a timeline before I meet them.

Once you put it on the timeline, you can see all the layers that are contributing to your symptoms – whether it be depression or not. I'm sure my list above is not complete, but these are the bulk of things I collect to figure out what my patients have been through, how they dealt with it, how resilient they were, when they were down, and how they got back up. Think about yourself and how you danced with your environment. Every interaction with the world is a dance. It's not nature or nurture. It's nature *and* nurture.

Look at how long these symptoms have been there and how they are connected. Where are your perfect storms? Circle the most recent one.

Write down every layer you have that might have contributed to that storm.

If you feel so inclined, circle a second or third one.

This is important so you can learn where your pain points or vulnerable areas of your life are and how to manage them in the maintenance phase in the future. It's important to develop an awareness of what they are and how they impact you daily.

Now we know the past and how it's contributing to how you feel.

What layers do you see that contributed to your perfect storm or storms? Write them all down in your journal. The purpose of doing this is to show you that multiple layers need to be addressed. I hope you can see that there is no way an antidepressant it going to take care of all of these issues. It might help in the beginning, but not likely in the long run. It is not a one-bullet approach.

Let's get an idea of how all of these issues have come together at this point. Complete the Multiple Symptom/Toxicity Questionnaire (MSQ) found at this link: https://drhyman. com/downloads/MSQ_Fillable.pdf. This is a questionnaire that tells you how toxic you are based on symptoms. It helps to identify the underlying causes of illness and to track them over time. The first time you fill it out, rate each symptom based on the last thirty days. After the first time, rate your symptoms in the last forty-eight hours only.

0	Never or almost never have the symptoms.
1	Occasionally have it, effect is not severe.
2	Occasionally have it, effect is severe.
3	Frequently have it, effect is not severe.
4	Frequently have it, effect is severe.

Some people have difficulty objectifying subjective feelings. *What matters most is that you are consistent in your thinking about these symptoms over time.* If you have the symptom, then rate it for frequency and intensity of distress.

We will use this to document your progress monthly, or weekly if you want, as you do my program as described in this book. As your symptoms improve, your score will drop.

Add individual scores and total each group. If you have a score of less than 10, that is optimal. However, if that score of 10 is within a particular category, then that can be a problem of focus. Mild toxicity is 10 to 50, moderate toxicity is 50 to 100 and severe toxicity is over 100. What causes this toxicity is rooted in inflammation through a variety of routes. If you follow the steps outlined in this book, you can follow your progress by completing the MSQ every month to see if it is effecting a change. It doesn't help to do it more often than that. The goal is to bring the score below 10, but ultimately, it is how you feel that is the true test. Completing this questionnaire is not necessary for you to continue reading the rest of this book.

By now, you might be a little overwhelmed but at least you've been able to bring to your awareness what the problems are. Believe it or not, having chronic constipation is a problem. Having PMS is a problem. Having a chronic runny nose is a problem. Passing smelly gas is a problem. Being one hundred pounds overweight is more socially acceptable, but it isn't healthy.

My experience is that the higher the score you have, the more you will gain from following the steps in the chapters to come. You could potentially feel significantly better in three months if you do all of the things noted in this book. At the end of Chapter 3, I provided a list of conditions that might take longer, barring some permanent irreversible injury.

To know what to do you need a destination, where you want to be in the future. When you decide to do a program, you want to have certain results and need to have the motivation to keep moving forward. You, yes, *you*, no one else, need to do some soul-searching and really think about where you want to be in order to decide how to get there. You can't plan a trip to a place until you pick the place first, right? Your plan to go to a tropical island is different from going to a ski resort. You have to pack differently and, depending on how long you're gone, you might need more than one suitcase. Do you get my drift? You would never get into a car and just drive or just hop on a plane for no reason or no planned destination. Other than a joyride, the likelihood is low. You will have a destination by completing the next exercise.

I would like you to complete the Perfect-Life Vision exercise I describe below. If it's too hard for you to look ten years ahead, you may change the time to seven or five years, even one year. This a right brain exercise to dream and be creative. You need a destination set in the future.

Write the answers in your journal:

1. It's ten years in the future and everything you've ever wanted to be, do, have, and experience has become a reality. The date is____________. Describe, in detail, everything that has happened over these past ten years to create your perfect life.

2. Why is this vision important to you?

3. Imagine you have everything you want and nothing is holding you back. What does your perfect day look like? Describe it from morning until night.

4. What does your life look like now?

5. What's standing in your way of living your perfect life? Make a list of obstacles, challenges, areas that are broken, or things that are missing.

6. What needs to happen, starting now, for you to overcome these challenges?

Once you come up with a vision, you can start to make micro-changes in your day to reach those goals noted in Question #3. This will hopefully motivate you to keep moving toward making your goals a reality. It's not set in stone and it can change. I learned about this exercise through Yuri Elkaim, an entrepreneur, holistic nutrition and fitness expert. I have since incorporated this exercise with many of my patients.

My hope is that, in this chapter, you will become more aware of what is happening in your body, and what's coursing through your mind. I would like you to become aware of the issues you've been struggling with, not only now, but likely for years, the ones you've just been living with, annoyed by, ignoring, or outright just didn't know were a problem. You can only change something after you've become aware of it. Then put the pieces of your puzzle together to find your perfect storm that caused your immune system to go on overload. Finally, choose a destination and create a plan of attack using the next four chapters. Sometimes people simply feel better just by figuring out the problem and having a plan. Feeling helpless and hopeless is a symptom that leads to depression; feeling empowered leads to healing.

CHAPTER 7

It Starts in the Gut

I mentioned in a previous chapter that when some people go to see their doctor, they might complain about fatigue, problems with sleep, or problems with concentration. Doctors might do a screening for depression and decide that the person is depressed and conclude that the physical symptoms are due to the depression. I hope I've convinced you that the physical symptoms are not necessarily caused by depression. The physical symptoms accompany the emotional symptoms of feeling sad, down, or apathetic. This combination of symptoms is most commonly called major depression or another type of depression called persistent depressive disorder, previously known as dysthymic disorder. It's a name to describe a cluster of symptoms. What is causing all of those symptoms? Enter inflammation. Most people don't quite understand what the immune system is or what inflammation is. Some people think that it's like a switch that is turned on or off. Far from that, it's a very complex system.

The way I describe the immune system is that it is like our military system. We have four branches of the immune system, IgA, IgG, IgM, and IgE. Just like the army, navy, marines, and air force, they have their roles in defending our country. Each branch has thousands of soldiers ready to be deployed and each branch has its method of attacking the enemy. Some catch the enemy to learn more about them. One branch tends to respond to specific threats based on where the threat is and sometimes these branches work together or in tandem. Even the local and state police have a concomitant system in the body.

It's not a perfect analogy, but our immune defense system is much like this on a cellular level. We have glucose to feed our immune cells, our blood system to transport the immune system to where it needs to go with oxygen, cholesterol to bind the enemy and clear away the trash in the repair phase, and cortisol to sound off the alarms and support the system.

Once the defense system has done its job and the threat is over, the next phase for the immune system is repair. This usually begins with firefighters and local police arriving at the scene to save people who can be saved and bring them to the hospital emergency rooms. Again, our body's repair system is not much different. It needs to be cared for so it can respond to daily stressors. It is constantly working.

One thing to know is that when there is a campaign to fight and defend, there is no repairing going on. The fight has to be over before the body can rebuild. If the house is on fire, the fire has to be put out before the house can be repaired. The maintenance crew steps out and the fire fighters rush in.

One part of the immune system can be dysfunctional and not be able to accomplish its job while another part of the immune system could be working optimally. Each part of the immune system has a specific job and is not likely to do the job of another part of the immune system. Your local police aren't likely to be deployed to a foreign country. That's why a person can have environmental allergies but not have an autoimmune disorder.

About seventy percent of the immune system is in the gut lining and that is the area in our body that directly interacts with the environment. The gut lining is only one-cell layer thick. It has a mucus layer on top and the immune system below examining everything as it goes by. It has a surveillance system to sample what is going through the gut. It's sort of like passing through customs. If you don't belong there, it will nab you, tag you, and take fingerprints. In the body, a cascade of triggers might cause the gates between these cells to open and induce a massive case of diarrhea to flush out the intruder. That intruder has to get past a lot of other checkpoints to even get that far. The stomach has an acid pit, and then the intruder is sprayed with enzymes and covered in bile to digest it. Those gates get stuck open for other reasons as well. Foods, toxins, and even stress can cause a leaky gut. Ideally, you want the gates to stay closed and only open when necessary. Imagine the gut lining like cheesecloth. When you wrap up spices in cheesecloth, only material broken down to the smallest pieces gets through. If there was a hole in the cheesecloth, then larger molecules will go through and trip an alarm. Food needs to be broken down to the point that it can get through without those gates being open. When these gates are open, the result is often inflammation. Our goal is to strengthen the immune system and close the gates.

An inflammatory response occurs in our body when the alarms are triggered that something has gone wrong or when there is a breakdown of our repair system.

Sometimes those gates open for good reason. When a baby is transitioning through the birth canal, its gates need to be open to receive its immune system from the mother. You obtain your immune system from your mother's birth canal and breast milk.

The processes of digestion are also two-fold: it sterilizes whatever we ingest to remove intruders (so we don't get sick) and breaks down our food into tiny bits so it can be assimilated.

Digestion begins in the brain. Have you ever opened up a food magazine and started to salivate? Smells, real or imagined, trigger the digestive process. Cooking the food "digests" it even further, then you cut it up in even smaller pieces on your plate. Chewing your food and mashing even more with your teeth makes it even smaller. This whole process is to break down food into pieces small enough to get through the cheesecloth-like one-cell layer thick lining of your gut. While you are chewing, you are lathering your food with saliva, which has enzymes to break it down even more. It goes down the esophagus, past the esophageal sphincter. The pH of the stomach shuts the sphincter. If that pH isn't low enough, the sphincter stays open. The stomach acid is hydrochloric acid (HCl), which is what is needed to break down protein, but it also sterilizes all of the food that passes through. Then the food gets past the pyloric sphincter and here the low pH of the acid shuts the sphincter behind it. The low pH of acid triggers the release of bile salts and pancreatic enzymes and also releases intrinsic factor to bind to Vitamin B12.

This orchestra of releasing digestive juices is necessary to break down the food you eat into individual proteins, fats, and carbohydrates. Once it crosses over to the other side of the gut lining, these raw materials get transported and assembled into the various materials the body needs. If you don't eat the right foods to provide those raw materials, then some things your body needs get made poorly or not at all. Imagine what happens when a house is being built and the supply of nails stops. The house either doesn't get built or those nails are substituted by cheaper ones. If the toilets don't get shipped, then parts of the house get built without the toilet. The toilets are added later. The body does the same thing. So life goes on, houses get built but cheaply or poorly.

A normal stomach acid level creates a pH of 1.5 to 2.5. As we age, the parietal cells in the stomach lining produce less hydrochloric acid (HCl). In fact, half of people over the age of sixty have hypochlorhydria (low stomach acid), and by age eighty-five, eighty percent of relatively healthy people have low stomach acid. Also, certain medications will affect stomach acid. Acid-blocking medications increase stomach pH to 3.5 or higher. This inhibits pepsin, which is a potential irritant to the stomach but is also essential for digestion of protein. Stomach acid is also necessary for absorption of many minerals. In addition, stomach acid provides our first defense against food poisoning, H. pylori, parasites, and other infections. Without adequate acid, we leave ourselves open to decreased immune resistance and a variety of other health problems. Overgrowth of bacteria in the small intestine occurs in twenty percent of people aged sixty to eighty and in forty percent of people over age eighty. Adequate HCl is necessary for the absorption of Vitamin B12 from food; B12 deficiency causes weakness, fatigue, and nervous system problems. Vitamin C levels are also low in people with poor stomach acid. Several minerals require an acidic environment for absorption, including iron, calcium, magnesium, zinc, and copper. Acid is critical for the breakdown of protein bonds in the stomach, and poor acid content in the stomach causes indigestion. The symptoms of hypoacidity often mimic those of hyperacidity.

Hypochlorhydria may be caused by the following: pernicious anemia, chronic H. pylori infection, long-term treatment with proton pump inhibitors (like Prilosec®), autoimmune gastritis, and mucolipidosis type IV.

Common Symptoms of Hypochlorhydria

- Bloating, belching, burning, and flatulence immediately after meals
- A sense of fullness after eating
- Indigestion, diarrhea, or constipation
- Multiple food allergies
- Nausea after taking supplements
- Itching around the rectum
- Weak, peeling, and cracked fingernails
- Dilated blood vessels in the cheeks and nose (in non-alcoholics)
- Acne
- Iron deficiency
- Chronic intestinal parasites or abnormal flora
- Undigested food in stool
- Chronic candida infections
- Upper digestive tract gassiness

Diseases Associated with Hypochlorhydria

- Addison's disease
- Asthma
- Celiac disease
- Chronic autoimmune disorders
- Chronic hives
- Dermatitis herpetiformis (gluten sensitivity)
- Diabetes
- Eczema
- Gallbladder disease

- Graves' disease
- Hepatitis
- Hyper- and hypothyroidism
- Lupus erythematosus
- Myasthenia gravis
- Osteoporosis
- Pernicious anemia
- Psoriasis
- Rheumatoid arthritis
- Rosacea
- Sjögren's syndrome
- Thyrotoxicosis
- Vitiligo

If you are on an acid-reducing medication, you may want to discuss with your provider about whether it is still appropriate for you to continue, especially if you have any of the above symptoms or conditions. The package insert indicates that these medications should not be taken long term unless you have specific conditions that warrant it, e.g., Zollinger-Ellison syndrome and Barrett's esophagus. Many people are misdiagnosed with acid reflux caused by too much acid when it's actually from not making enough acid. Some hospitals' staff start patients on proton pump inhibitors on admission to prevent stress ulcers whether or not they have symptoms and fail to discontinue them upon discharge.

The Institute for Functional Medicine recommends self-testing by doing a betaine HCl Challenge the following way.

Self-Testing and Treatment for Low HCl (Hypochlorhydria)

1. Begin by taking one 350-750 mg capsule of Betaine HCl with a protein-containing meal.
   - A normal response in a healthy person would be discomfort – basically heartburn.
   - If you do not feel a burning sensation, begin taking two capsules with each protein-containing meal.

2. If there are no reactions after two days, increase the number of capsules with each meal to three.

3. Continue increasing the number of capsules every two days, using up to five capsules (or as your healthcare professional suggests) with each meal if necessary.
   - These dosages may seem large, but a normally functioning stomach manufactures considerably more.
   - You'll know you've taken too much if you experience tingling, heartburn, diarrhea, or any type of discomfort including a feeling of unease, digestive discomfort, neck ache, backache, headache, or any new odd symptom.
   - If you experience tingling, burning, or any symptom that is uncomfortable, you can neutralize the acid with one teaspoon of baking soda in water or milk.

4. When you reach a state of tingling, burning, or any other type of discomfort, cut back by one capsule per meal. If the discomfort continues, discontinue the HCl and consult with your healthcare professional.

5. Once you have established a dose (up to five capsules) that causes no symptoms, continue until your next appointment.

6. With smaller meals, you may require less HCl so you may reduce the amount of capsules taken. Individuals with a mild HCl deficiency may regain some normal HCl secretion and thus may over time have some symptoms of heartburn from taking the HCl. Simply decrease the number of capsules you are taking until the symptoms disappear. Individuals with moderate to severely low HCl/pepsin typically do not experience such quick improvement, so to maximize the absorption and benefits of the nutrients taken, it is important to be consistent with HCl supplementation.

Precautions: *Administration of HCl/pepsin is contraindicated in peptic ulcer disease. HCl can irritate sensitive tissue and can be corrosive to teeth; therefore, capsules should not be emptied into food or dissolved in beverages. Always follow up with your health care provider in four to six weeks or if you have any questions. Used with permission from The Institute for Functional Medicine (IFM), the global leader in Functional Medicine and a collaborator in the transformation of healthcare. IFM is a 501(c)(3) nonprofit organization that believes Functional Medicine can help every individual reach their full potential for health and well-being. Under no circumstances may the whole or any part of the materials be translated into another language, nor may you create derivative or other works without IFM's prior written permission (for permission please contact info@ifm.org).*

My preference is to do the baking soda stomach acid test to be sure that the stomach is not making enough hydrochloric acid, as I feel that it's a precaution against potentially causing gastritis. In my early days of doing functional medicine, an eighteen-year-old patient ended up having gastritis because he didn't do the baking soda test that I describe below and just started to take Betaine HCl. I always caution my younger patients to treat it as a jumpstarting of their gastric flow rather than actually needing it long term – like what you might have to do if you store your car over the winter and can't turn it over. Younger people might just need a jumpstart with only a few days to a week of taking this type of supplement.

The baking soda (Sodium Bicarbonate) solution reacts with the acid in the stomach to produce carbon dioxide. Think volcano experiment. $HCl + NaHCO_3$ (baking soda) reacts and becomes $NaCl + H_2O + CO_2$ (carbon dioxide gas) The amount of gas produced depends upon the quantity of acid contained in the stomach. Carry out the following steps to determine your stomach acidity:

1. Perform this test first thing in the morning on an empty stomach, before eating or drinking (before taking medications for heartburn).

2. Dissolve ¼ teaspoon of baking soda (make sure it's fresh) into an eight ounce glass of cold water.

3. Drink the solution and record the start time.

4. Record the time until you first burp up gas.

5. Perform this test for four consecutive days (or longer) at the same time each day, in order to give a better estimation of your stomach's acidity. It is not the most accurate test, which is why it should be repeated. Sometimes people swallow air and confuse that with a burp. However, burping repeatedly and loudly could indicate too much stomach acid. I have my patients report their experience and results to me before starting betaine HCl with pepsin.

Day	Time (min) until First Burp
1.	
2.	
3.	
4.	

Use this scale to determine what the result means.

< 2 minutes	normal acidity
2-5 minutes	low-normal acidity
> 5 minutes	probable hypochlorhydria (if you find that you are at low normal burping)

Depending on the results, then you may begin taking two tablespoons of apple cider vinegar, mixing it in eight ounces of water, and drinking this mixture fifteen minutes before your meals. Get an unfiltered brand like Bragg's Organic Raw; you'll get the added benefits of the probiotics it contains. This will stimulate production of HCl. Some people like to use bitters before meals to stimulate acid production. If you find that this is not enough, you may need Betaine HCl if you aren't burping at all.

The two tests above are tests you can do in your home. The Heidelberg Stomach Acid Test is a test that is the gold standard for testing of stomach acid production. It costs about $350 and insurance generally will not pay for it. You have to fast for twelve hours, then swallow a capsule with a radio transmitter in it, which then records the pH of your stomach as you drink a solution with sodium bicarbonate in it. It will print out a graph that shows your pH levels over time. I personally have been satisfied with the baking soda test. However, I wouldn't hesitate to use the Heidelberg Stomach Acid Test if I received inconclusive results.

Not only is it important to choose the proper foods, it is equally important to make sure that the food is being digested and assimilated into the body. The main function of the small intestine is the absorption of nutrients and minerals. Eighty percent of digestion occurs in the small intestine, ten percent occurs in the stomach, and ten percent occurs in the large intestine.

The large intestine is basically a large dishwasher and a trash compactor. The fiber in the food you eat is broken down into soluble fiber and insoluble fiber. We eat fiber to move things along and clean the inside of our intestines. Fiber is like one of those yellow sponges with the green scrubby part used to clean the dishes. Soluble fiber is like the yellow part of the sponge and the insoluble fiber is like the green part. Much of the insoluble fiber becomes the bulk of your stool. The rest of your stool is all the trash dumped into your bloodstream by your organs that was filtered out by your liver. Some trash is breathed out by your lungs and some trash is urinated out through your kidneys. It's extremely important to put out the trash. You know what happens if the trash stays in your trash can for too long? It begins to smell and maybe seep into other things. The same happens in the body; it does seep into your other organs and causes another form of toxicity or inflammation. All your organs are pressed up against each other.

Having bowel movements daily (or ideally several times a day) is important. There is a rhythm or conveyor belt to move things along. When a person eats, a gastrocolic reflex gets triggered. It's the body's way of telling the large intestine to make room. There are some foods that trigger it more quickly than others and some people have a more sensitive gastrocolic reflex. The larger the meal and the higher the fat and fiber content, the stronger the reflex will be.

Evaluating the consistency and timing of bowel movements tells us a lot about what is going on in the body. You can get a Bowel Movement Record form, which is an adaptation of the Bristol Stool Form Scale, at this link: https://www.nhsggc.org.uk/media/241191/nhsggc-bristol-stool-chart.pdf.

Generally, you will want to have a bowel movement that looks like a snake and isn't difficult to pass. You can look at the Bristol Stool Form Scale; ideally you will want your bowel movements to be Type 4, but having variations between Types 3 to 5 is acceptable. It shouldn't require lots of toilet paper. In fact, using a lot of toilet paper is a sign that you might have dysbiosis, an imbalance of the gut microbiome.

One of the most common health hazards and problems in Western civilization is chronic constipation and disease of the colon, e.g., hemorrhoids, diverticulitis, colitis, cancer of the colon, and auto-toxicity (self-poisoning) from chronic constipation.

Studies of other cultures have consistently shown the correlation between healthy colons, large stools, and normal colon transit time. African and Asian natives from rural communities who eat bulky, high-fiber diets with little or no meat and no refined foods have almost no heart disease, atherosclerosis, cancer (especially of the colon and rectum), diabetes, appendicitis, mental disease, and hypoglycemia.

In addition to the consistency and frequency of bowel movements, a measure of colon health is the colon transit time. This is done simply by eating a moderate serving of corn or beets or taking activated charcoal capsules and observing their appearance in the stool.

Directions

1. Consume a moderate serving (1/2 to 3/4 cup) of corn or beets or four charcoal capsules.

   Date: _________________ Exact Time:_________________

2. Visually examine stool (bowel movements), and note when corn or beets or charcoal are *first* seen. (Beets are seen as a redness in stool color, charcoal will turn the stool black, and corn is seen as whole corn.)

   Date: _________________ Exact Time:_________________

3. Note time when corn or beets or charcoal are *last* seen in stool.

   Date: _________________ Exact Time:_________________

4. On a typical day, how often do you move your bowels and are they formed or loose or somewhere in between? Please describe.

   ____

   ____

The time between when you ingested the corn, beets, or charcoal to the time it first appears in your stool and stops appearing in your stool is your bowel transit time range. People who live in rural African and Asian societies have a colon transit time of between twelve to twenty-four hours. In our American culture, the average colon transit time is much longer. A long transit time indicates suboptimal colon health. A fast transit time indicate poor absorption and assimilation of nutrients. Both conditions need to be corrected.

Note: Used with permission from The Institute for Functional Medicine (IFM), the global leader in Functional Medicine and a collaborator in the

The types of foods you eat and how much fluid you drink are key factors. There is variation in transit time within an individual and between people. People who eat more vegetables, fruit, and whole grains tend to have a quicker transit time than people who eat mostly sugars and starches.

Hypermobility means that food moves too quickly through your gastrointestinal tract. If this happens, you may be at risk of nutrient deficiencies because there is less absorption time. When it's too fast, you can get dehydrated, have electrolyte imbalances, and low levels of vitamins and minerals that affect skin health, hair health, energy level, and more. A transit time less of than twelve hours might indicate a malabsorption problem.

Hypomobility means that the food is moving too slowly, and the stool sits inside your colon for too long. Slow transit time increases the risk of colon disease. When that happens, the trash or waste products carried out of the liver in bile or from our food can get absorbed back into the system where they can irritate and/or inflame your system. Again, roughly speaking, a transit time of more than about twenty-four hours may indicate a slow transit time.

Some of the reasons why your transit time may be too fast can be from medication side effects, bacterial overgrowth from the colon into the small bowel producing gas that then speeds up transit time (hydrogen producing microbes), other bacterial or parasitic infections, supplements, and the fight-or-flight response of stress.

Some of the reasons why it might be too slow, include bacterial overgrowth from the colon into the small bowel producing gas that slows down transit time (methane producing microbes), Parkinson's disease, hypothyroidism, or delayed gastric emptying (stomach is slower than normal to release into the small intestine). The inflammatory diseases such as ulcerative colitis or Crohn's disease can cause either.

Just evaluating the entire process of digestion and correcting wherever it needs to be corrected can support and strengthen the immune system as well as improve absorption and assimilation of nutrients. If you were running a factory, you would check that all systems are working before blaming the workers for not doing their jobs.

There are many things that can disrupt this process and cause mental health and physical symptoms. The vagus nerve (cranial nerve X) is intimately connected to the gut. Sometimes this nerve can be shocked by events like a concussion or even repeated minor injuries like hitting a soccer ball with your head. When this happens, the gut shuts down, peristalsis stops, and the whole manufacturing system slows. Stress can trigger the sympathetic system that inhibits the parasympathetic system of resting and digesting. The sympathetic system is the system that makes you fight, flight, freeze, faint, or be appeased. The parasympathetic system is in charge of resting and digesting. The brain influences the gut and vice versa. Some have called the gut the second brain. The microbiome is a community of bacteria that utilize the nutrients to make what our bodies need. They are the workers in our factories and the soldiers of our immune system.

Many people rush around in their daily lives eating on the run, in the car or in front of the computer wolfing down their food. Some people have a poor relationship with food or none at all. Most people eat for pleasure or to shut down hunger pains, not as a source of sustenance - as medicine to heal and repair the machinery within. Generally, people don't think about what they are putting into their bodies. They take it for granted. Think about how long a car or home would last if it was maintained the same way. Many people, doctors even, look at food as calories in and calories out.

There are two other systems in the body that very few people talk about – that being the endocannabinoid system and the lymphatic system. The endocannabinoid system is intimately connected to your gut and brain. When we react to stress, this system tones down and modulates the Hypothalamic Pituitary Adrenal (HPA) axis to protect us from stress. This, in turn, signals the GI system to calm down. The second system is the lymphatic system. Lymph is the fluid that your body collects from interstitial fluid, the fluid that lies between cells. It's designed to return dead cells, proteins, and excess interstitial fluid back to the circulation system for removal. Lymph helps to remove some bacteria, cancerous cells, and toxic metabolites. It also transports fats from the digestive system.

After making sure the digestive processes are evaluated and supported, it is important to address the sources of inflammation in connection to the gut and do the Five R program of gut restoration – Remove, Replace, Re-inoculate, Repair, and Rebalance. Other chapters will go into detail with each of these areas. We want to remove things to SHIFT your physiology. SHIFT just happens to be a great acronym to remember what they are: stress, hormones, infections, foods, and toxins.

By *removing* these things, we will reduce inflammation and put out the metaphorical fire so that the body can start repairing. Then we will *replace* what's been missing by providing health foods and other nutrients by other means. I provide supplements as a bridge to health to get the body back to a place where it's functioning; until the person can make lifestyle and dietary changes to meet their needs. However, some people have genetic SNPs, or single nucleotide polymorphisms, which are genes that work less efficiently and therefore result in the need for long-term use of supplements. Others can't or don't want to make certain dietary changes. We might replace hormones when needed. We then *re-inoculate* the gut microbiome with probiotics. These days there are numerous different types of probiotics – different spectrums and dosages. Sometimes I give soil-based probiotics or certain species for specific conditions. Since probiotics affect a change but don't hang around for very long, I like to give short-chain fatty acids like butyrate and propionate to feed the gut microbiome. Then the next phase is *repair* – to supply the ingredients to heal the gut lining – the mucous layer above and the immune system below, and to close the gates causing permeability. This is a phase that some practitioners don't do because the patient feels so good, they drop out of treatment. Symptoms return when they go back to their old lifestyle. It might also be forgotten because the patient feels so good and is stuck in a restricted mode of living. It's very important to do this phase and then *reintroduce* foods back into the diet carefully.

Last but not least, I want to talk about rhythms.

We are part of an ecosystem. We're on this swirling planet affected by the phases of the moon that takes a year to travel around the sun. We are aware on a daily basis of the rising and falling of the sun and the moon. Most people usually don't notice that the rising slowly moves across the horizon. I have a beautiful view of the sunrise from my bed, through the trees and in the course of the year, I watch it move from all of the way to the left to all of the way to the right. These shifts are perceptible in the course of a week. Walking on the beach, one might be connected to the tides – when they come in and when they go out.

Animals are intimately connected to the land and to each other. Humans really are the same way. I went to an experiential conference and they had us do an exercise. We were asked to walk in any direction and continue walking randomly without bumping into anyone else. Then we were asked to silently pair up with someone and walk together. We had to communicate with our movements in relation to each other and walk together. Who knew who was leading? How did we communicate that? Something interesting happened while we were all focused on only one other person. We spontaneously fell into all moving in one gigantic circle.

We as humans have lost this connection. Most of us stare at a phone. We've lost our rhythms. We used to have rituals that connected to these rhythms, that connected to each other and to ourselves on a daily basis, not just once a week in a church, temple, or mosque, but in our homes, alone with ourselves and with our families.

Our circadian rhythms are entrained with the sun, specifically to blue light, and when the sun goes down, our melatonin production goes up. Blue light suppresses melatonin production and promotes wakefulness.

With the advent of electricity and with the types of lighting we are exposed to, we don't go to sleep when the sun goes down. If you work at night and sleep during the day, research has shown that the graveyard shift takes twenty years off your life. Sleep is the time that the repair processes in our body happen and research shows that the hours of eleven p.m. to two a.m. are the most critical hours. One cannot shift those hours to your schedule. The body is resilient, and it can handle being awake during those hours, but there is a cost. Some people are stuck on getting eight hours of sleep, while there are some people who are fine with five hours of sleep and others that need ten hours. How much sleep you need is dependent on your activity level. If you sit around all day and do nothing, you won't need to sleep that much. To determine how much sleep you need, think about a stable period of time in your life when you slept well and felt rested upon awakening. That's the number of hours you should shoot for. Ultimately, it's feeling rested upon awakening that is the key to knowing how much sleep you need. Your requirements for sleep will change over your lifetime. Most people dream, so if you don't dream or have no dream recall, that is an indication that you may be deficient in Vitamin B6.

I make these types of recommendations to improve your sleep. Go through each one to make sure you are doing them.

- Avoid caffeine, alcohol, nicotine, and other chemicals that interfere with sleep.

- Go to bed at the same time every night and wake up at the same time every morning. It's the wake-up time that sets your biological clock.

- Ease the transition from wake time to sleep time with a period of relaxing activities an hour or so before bed. Take a bath (the rise then fall in body temperature promotes drowsiness), read a book, watch television, or practice relaxation exercises. Avoid stressful, stimulating activities like doing work or discussing emotional issues.

- Turn your bedroom into a sleep-inducing environment

– dark cool place, use earplugs or white noise, and sleep on a comfortable mattress. Remove the TV from the room. Use your bed just for sleep and sex.

- Turn your clock's face away from you and if you wake up in the middle of the night and can't get back to sleep in about twenty minutes, get up and engage in a quiet, restful activity such as reading or listening to music. And keep the lights dim; as bright light can stimulate your internal clock. When your eyelids are drooping and you are ready to sleep, return to bed.

- Many people make naps a regular part of their day. However, for those who find falling asleep or staying asleep through the night problematic, afternoon napping may be one of the culprits. This is because late-day naps decrease sleep drive. If you must nap, it's better to keep it short and before five p.m.

- Finish dinner several hours before bedtime and avoid foods that cause indigestion. If you get hungry at night, snack on foods that (in your experience) won't disturb your sleep, perhaps dairy foods and carbohydrates.

- Drink enough fluid at night to keep from waking up thirsty – but not so much and so close to bedtime that you will be awakened by the need for a trip to the bathroom.

- If you wake up with a dry mouth, consider taping your mouth shut. That is, if you can breathe through your nose – if you can't, get that evaluated. Mouth breathing is problematic for many reasons.

- Exercise can help you fall asleep faster and sleep more

soundly – as long as it's done at the right time. Exercise stimulates the body to secrete the stress hormone cortisol, which helps activate the alerting mechanism in the brain. This is fine unless you're trying to fall asleep. Try to finish exercising at least three hours before bed or work out earlier in the day.

- Fluorescent and LED lighting expose you to a lot of blue light. Computers and phones can cause you to stay up at night. If you have to work at night on the computer, try the free download from https://justgetflux.com/. It's called f.lux, and it makes the color of your computer's display adapt to the time of day, warm lighting at night and bright like sunlight during the day. f.lux may help you sleep better.

I had a patient move into a densely populated area and found that she wasn't sleeping. She discovered that she was sleeping near a bank of smart meters emitting EMFs. As a result, she was forced to move and was able to sleep well again. Anything that creates microwave radiation like Wi-Fi routers and "smart appliances" should be turned off, especially if they are near the bedroom.

Some of these tips will be easier to include in your daily and nightly routine than others. However, if you stick with them, your chances of achieving restful sleep will improve. That said, not all sleep problems are easily treated and could signify the presence of a sleep disorder such as apnea, restless legs syndrome, narcolepsy, or another clinical sleep problem. If your sleep difficulties don't improve through good sleep hygiene, this would be something to discuss with your primary care provider for a thorough evaluation.

Here are some apps to help you sleep:

- CBTI-Coach: https://mobile.va.gov/app/cbt-i-coach
- SleepRate: https://www.sleeprate.com/apps/
- Sleepio: https://www.sleepio.com/
- Go! to Sleep: https://my.clevelandclinic.org/mobile-apps/go-to-sleep-app
- Sleep Cycle: https://www.sleepcycle.com/how-sleep-cycle-works/

I like these apps because they keep you on track and record your progress. The information can then be shared with others.

Another type of rhythm is movement. We don't move enough - period. Most of us – young and old – sit in a chair in front of a screen. I dislike exercise but I love team sports. I play ultimate frisbee during three seasons but sitting all day long actually has impeded my performance, so I try to find ways to incorporate movement into my daily life. I've gotten a standing desk and a Gaiam ball chair (https://www.gaiam.com/products/classic-balance-ball-chair) and it made a huge difference in improving my Achilles pain. My husband exercises like a robot. It's funny because he is actually a roboticist. But anyway, he gets up every morning, gets on his stationary bike, and rides it while watching the sunrise and lifting little hand weights. Then in the evening, he gets on the elliptical followed by a yoga routine. I don't know how he does it. Most people are not that regimented. Honestly, you don't need to be. I'm not. Just find ways to move.

Movement is important because it activates and improves your immune system unless you overdo it. The process of hormesis is when low doses of external stressors that are noxious at higher levels can benefit cells. In fact, hormesis turns on and off genes related to maintenance and repair pathways in your body. Moderate exercise is enough to make these changes and support the immune system.

Just walking briskly fifteen to thirty minutes daily is the minimum you need to do to support the process of healing. When going from place to place, park a distance from your intended destination to work in some walking. Try to walk at a quicker pace if you can.

Research has shown that doing a seven-minute high-intensity interval training workout daily is all you need to boost your immune system. The goal overall is to raise your heart rate in short bursts. Just Google "NY Times 7-Minute Workout" or click on this link: https://well.blogs.nytimes.com/2013/05/09/the-scientific-7-minute-workout/. You can download an app on your phone by the same name. You want to make sure you are able to do all of the movements safely, so watch the video first. If not, do a variation of it.

If you choose walking, when you walk, you can boost your immune system by increasing your pace for thirty seconds every five minutes to increase your heart rate and respiration. You can take breaks and walk up and down the stairwells with a co-worker.

I like to dance and sing in my house or in the shower, so I turn on my favorite three songs and dance to them. My current favorites are *Cheap Thrills* by Sia, *Uptown Funk* by Mark Ronson feat. Bruno Mars, and *Party Rock Anthem* by LMFAO. When these songs are playing, I can't *not* dance or just even move a little to the music. I play these songs in the morning when I wake up and they get me awake and out of bed sometimes. Have you ever been to a wedding and ran onto the dance floor and thought, *I can't miss this one*? If dancing is not for you, think about what *is* for you. What did you do as a child or a teenager and how could you fit those activities back into your life on some level? Or think about what activity you'd be interested in learning. If you are not a physical person but want to improve your flexibility and learn something you could use as you get older to extend your life, try learning a gentle form of yoga, tai chi, or qi gong.

Certainly, joining a gym or doing a team sport can take it to the next level, but the point is that it's not necessary. Remember, overdoing it can also set you back.

A type of movement that helps the immune system sync with itself is repetitive and bilateral movement. There are parts of us always moving – our breath and our heartbeat. Movement begins when an infant moves its arms up and down and then starts to crawl, alternating those movements. That crawling motion sends a signal to the brain that influences neural patterns of development. I caution people to not force babies to walk before their time. Twirling and rocking back and forth can be very healing. Drumming on your lap, playing patty-cake with another person, or tapping on your head and face sends signals to your brain that cross over from one side to the other, like a pendulum, and tells your body that you are present and you are safe. It tells the immune system that it can calm down and turn off the alarms. Even the resonance of sounds and guttural movements of the throat can be healing. My favorite part of doing yoga is saying three "OMs" together with fifty people. The vibrations and synchronicity of the sound can run deep into your soul. It's a way of connecting and being separate at the same time. It causes movement on a cellular level.

Hippocrates said, "All disease begins in the gut." Maybe there is a reason why people say, "Go with your gut." The gut is our second brain, but the more I learn about it, I wonder if our first brain started with the microbiota – a community in our gut weighing four point five pounds containing tens of trillions of microorganisms, including over a thousand different species of known bacteria with more than three million genes (which is one hundred and fifty times more than human genes).

CHAPTER 8

Invisible Hijackers

I mentioned in a previous chapter that we are unraveling the biochemistry and SHIFTing the physiology of your body to eliminate symptoms that are telling you that your body is out of balance. And we do this by bringing your body back into balance or homeostasis. Thus, we'll start with handling the I in SHIFT, for Infections.

Most people think of infections as something that comes on quickly, makes you feel bad for a few days, and might give you a temperature, which means it's time to go to the doctor. The doctor might tell you to take Tylenol, which I would caution against because it inhibits your body's ability to mount a healthy defense against the infection and, more importantly, even one dose depletes your body's primary antioxidant, glutathione. Tylenol is best to use when your temperature is too high and unremitting, when the body is weakening and unable to mount a defense. You might also be given an antibiotic and, after a few days, feel better and think it's completely gone. What you don't know is what is happening at the level of the micro-organism.

Nowadays, and for good reason, doctors are catching on to the idea of not over-prescribing antibiotics. Doctors might wait a few days, as the condition might be viral, or they might culture the area of infection to help choose the narrowest of spectrums of antibiotics for treatment.

Antibiotics have saved countless lives. They were an easy fix and given often, but then we learned about antibiotic resistance like MRSA, which is methicillin-resistant staph aureus. People began dying from bacteria that no antibiotic could eradicate. So now, some antibiotics are reserved for certain situations so that bacteria cannot develop a resistance to it.

It was only recently that we've learned what antibiotics have done to our microbiome. I equate a round of antibiotics to a microbiome atomic bomb. An antibiotic kills almost everything – the bad guys and the good guys. People might have had a beneficial family of bacteria in their gut that will never return. Fortunately, seeds of those bacteria grow just like trees and plants grew again in Nagasaki or Hiroshima. What grows back is based on what you eat to feed those bacteria. The good bacteria that strengthen our immune system and help our bodies want vegetables, mostly green vegetables but ideally a rainbow color of vegetables. Vegetables are preferable for the growth of a diverse microbiome as they affect the most change as compared to other categories of food.

Sometimes there is a stalemate between your immune system and the foreign entity that is occupying their terrain. Although the bulk of the immune system is in the gut, you need to know that there are bacteria all over you, inside-and-out to protect you. That might skeeve you out, but if you didn't have a microbiome, you would need to live in a bubble. Anything unnatural that you put in or on your body, your immune system has to deal with day in and day out. Remember the rain barrel I mentioned in a previous chapter? When you put on that suntan lotion, you are killing the bacteria that is part of your immune system and then adding toxins to your body that is burdening your immune system to remove it. Not only is it doing that, it is also killing the coral reefs in Hawaii. (Hawaii recently banned suntan lotion because of it.)

Getting back to the stalemate, there are compromises made between countries like India and Pakistan. They might not like each other but they must put up with each other. Sometimes in the body, there are stalemates between our bacteria and other bacteria that don't belong in certain parts of the body. They might belong to another part of the body like the mouth but end up in the gut because certain barriers were compromised. Those barriers could be compromised by stress, inflammatory foods, or toxins. Taking steroids is sometimes lifesaving, but it compromises your immune system and allows pathogens to invade because steroids turn off your immune system. There might be bacteria that don't belong in the body at all. Then there are other pathogens like viruses, parasites, and worms that can also take up residence.

A clue for chronic infection is having repeated bouts of the same infections, for example, throat infections, chronic bronchitis, colitis, cellulitis, and urinary tract infections. Another clue is if you've had a really bad infection, for example food poisoning or after an area of the body has been breached, for example, surgery, and just never felt the same again. For example, I had a patient who had his wisdom teeth taken out and had a reaction to the pain medications, causing him to throw up and infect the wound. It's this type of information I look for in creating a timeline.

Sinus infections, root canals, and mouth infections are a major source of chronic infections in the gut.

When a person takes antibiotics, the antibiotics kill the bacteria that causes the infection but they also wipe out the good bacteria. If and when that happens, it's best to concurrently take probiotics that include Saccromyces boulardii, a good yeast to prevent yeast overgrowth and eat good sources of food to grow back the microbiome to a healthy population. If you eat unhealthy food, then the micro-organisms that have survived will thrive especially since the good bacteria are no longer present in quantities to keep them in check. One category of micro-organisms is yeast. Yeast is part of our normal flora and it's the good bacteria that keep these guys in check. When the bacteria are out of town because of chronic use or repeated use of antibiotics, yeast takes over and flourishes in an environment bathed in alcohol, sugar, processed food, and stress and thrive in people who take NSAIDs, BCP, and steroids including inhalers. They are a major cause of sugar cravings and cravings for bread. If you've ever had a yeast infection after taking antibiotics or had jock itch or genital itch, then you have likely had Candida. There are other types of yeast infections, but Candida is the most common.

My husband had a bout of acute prostatitis while we were in France. When we returned home, he saw a urologist who treated it repeatedly with antibiotics. He was led to believe that he would have to deal with intermittent infections and pain for the rest of his life. Fortunately, after my training at the IFM, I realized that what he had was chronic prostatitis because of yeast overgrowth. While we were in India, we all took doxycycline as a preventative for malaria. I gave him three months of antifungals. The symptoms completely remitted and he never had another bout again.

Unfortunately, there are many doctors who "don't believe in Candida" or call it a myth because they understand it to be part of the normal flora. They think that only people with HIV or people who are severely immunocompromised get this. It's not so black and white. Think about it as a garden. Weeds can be kept in check by changing the environment to make it hard for them to take root. However, once they take root, they can take over in a menacing way.

When Candida is given the opportunity to take over, it does on a pathologic level – just like normal average everyday people might join a mob in progress or loot a store when there is chaos in a society, but are law-abiding citizens when there is structured society.

Complete this questionnaire to see whether Candida might be a factor for you. For each section, read the directions and score as indicated. Total your score and record it at the end of the section. Add the totals for each section to get your Grand Total Score.

For each "yes" answer, circle the point score for that question. Add up the total score and record it at the end of this section.

Questions in Section A focus on your medical history – factors that promote the growth of Candida albicans and that are frequently found in people with yeast-related health problems.

In Section B you'll find a list of twenty-three symptoms that are often present in patients with yeast-related health problems.

Section C consists of thirty-three other symptoms that are sometimes seen in people with yeast-related problems – yet they also may be found in people with other disorders.

Filling out and scoring this questionnaire should help you and your physician evaluate the possible role Candida albicans contributes to your health problems. Naturally, it will not provide an automatic "yes" or "no" answer.

Section A: History

Section A: History		Point Score
1. Have you taken tetracyclines (Sumycin, Panmycino, Vibramycin, Minocin, etc.) or other antibiotics for acne for 1 month (or longer)?		35
2. Have you at any time in your life taken "broad spectrum" antibiotics* or other antibacterial medication for respiratory, urinary or other infections for two months or longer, or in shorter courses four or more times in a one-year period?		35
3. Have you taken a broad-spectrum antibiotic drug* – even in a single dose?		6
4. Have you, at any time in your life, been bothered by persistent prostatitis, vaginitis or other problems affecting your reproductive organs?		25
5. Have you been pregnant?	*One time?*	3
	Two or more times?	5
6. Have you taken birth control pills?	*For six months to two years?*	8
	For more than two years?	15
7. Have you taken prednisone, decadron or other cortisone-type drugs?	*For two weeks or less?*	6
	For more than two weeks?	15

Section A: History		Point Score
8. Does exposure to perfumes, insecticides, fabric shop odors, and other chemicals provoke symptoms?	*Mild symptoms?*	5
	Moderate to severe symptoms?	20
9. Are your symptoms worse on damp, muggy days or in moldy places?		20
10. Have you had athlete's foot, ringworm, "jock itch," or other chronic fungus infections of the skin or nails?	*Mild to moderate?*	10
	Severe or persistent?	20
11. Do you crave sugar?		10
12. Do you crave breads?		10
13. Do you crave alcoholic beverages?		10
14. Does tobacco smoke really bother you?		10
SECTION A TOTAL		

Section B: Major Symptoms

Section B: Major Symptoms	Point Score		
	Occasional and/or Mild	Frequent and/or Moderately Severe	Very Frequent and/or Very Severe or Disabling
1. Fatigue or lethargy	3	6	9
2. Feeling of being "drained"	3	6	9
3. Poor memory	3	6	9
4. Depression	3	6	9
5. Feeling "spacey" or "unreal"	3	6	9
6. Inability to make decisions	3	6	9
7. Numbness, burning, or tingling	3	6	9
8. Muscle aches or weakness	3	6	9
9. Pain and/or swelling in joints	3	6	9
10. Abdominal pain	3	6	9
11. Constipation	3	6	9
12. Diarrhea	3	6	9
13. Bloating, belching, or intestinal gas	3	6	9
14. Troublesome vaginal burning, itching, or discharge	3	6	9

Section B: Major Symptoms	Point Score		
	Occasional and/or Mild	Frequent and/or Moderately Severe	Very Frequent and/or Very Severe or Disabling
15. Persistent vaginal burning or itching	3	6	9
16. Prostatitis	3	6	9
17. Impotence	3	6	9
18. Loss of sexual desire or feeling	3	6	9
19. Endometriosis or infertility	3	6	9
20. Cramps and/or other menstrual irregularities	3	6	9
21. Premenstrual tension	3	6	9
22. Attacks of anxiety or crying	3	6	9
23. Cold hands or feet and/or chilliness	3	6	9
24. Shaking or irritable when hungry	3	6	9
SECTION B TOTAL			

Section C: Other Symptoms*

Section C: Other Symptoms	Point Scores		
	Occasional and/or Mild	Frequent and/or Moderately Severe	Very Frequent and/or Very Severe or Disabling
1. Drowsiness	1	2	3
2. Irritability or jitteriness	1	2	3
3. Incoordination	1	2	3
4. Inability to concentrate	1	2	3
5. Frequent mood swings	1	2	3
6. Headache	1	2	3
7. Dizziness/loss of balance	1	2	3
8. Pressure above ears, feeling of head swelling	1	2	3
9. Tendency to bruise easily	1	2	3
10. Chronic rashes or itching	1	2	3
11. Numbness, tingling	1	2	3
12. Indigestion or heartburn	1	2	3
13. Food sensitivity or intolerance	1	2	3
14. Mucus in stools	1	2	3
15. Rectal itching	1	2	3
16. Dry mouth or throat	1	2	3
17. Rash or blisters in mouth	1	2	3
18. Bad breath	1	2	3

Section C: Other Symptoms	Point Scores		
	Occasional and/or Mild	Frequent and/or Moderately Severe	Very Frequent and/or Very Severe or Disabling
19. Foot, body, or hair odor not relieved by washing	1	2	3
20. Nasal congestion or postnasal drip	1	2	3
21. Nasal itching	1	2	3
22. Sore throat	1	2	3
23. Laryngitis, loss of voice	1	2	3
24. Cough or recurrent bronchitis	1	2	3
25. Pain or tightness in chest	1	2	3
26. Wheezing or shortness of breath	1	2	3
27. Urgency or urinary frequency	1	2	3
28. Burning on urination	1	2	3
29. Spots in front of eyes or erratic vision	1	2	3
30. Burning or tearing of eyes	1	2	3
31. Recurrent infections or fluid in ears	1	2	3
32. Ear pain or deafness	1	2	3
SECTION C TOTAL			

Section A Total Score ________________

Section B Total Score ________________

Section C Total Score ________________

Grand Total Score ________________

The Grand Total Score will help you and your clinician decide if your health problems are yeast-connected. Scores in women will run higher, as seven items in the questionnaire apply exclusively to women, while only two apply exclusively to men.

Men	Women	Interpretation
40 or below	60 or below	Yeast is less apt to cause health problems
41-90	61-121	Yeast-connected health problems are possibly present
91-140	121-180	Yeast-connected health problems are probably present
141 or higher	181 or higher	Yeast-connected health problems are almost certainly present

Note: Used with permission from The Institute for Functional Medicine (IFM), the global leader in Functional Medicine and a collaborator in the transformation of healthcare. IFM is a 501(c)(3) nonprofit organization that believes Functional Medicine can help every individual reach their full potential for health and well-being. Under no circumstances may the whole or any part of the materials be translated into another language, nor may you create derivative or other works without IFM's prior written permission (for permission please contact info@ifm.org).

This yeast is a bugger to manage, but what you need to know is that this is a major cause of many symptoms. And the best way to figure out if this is a factor involved in your symptoms besides the questionnaire is to do a urine microbial organic acid test. Great Plains Laboratory (https://www.greatplainslaboratory.com/) performs this test for less than $250.

If you have a tough time controlling your sugar intake, it feels like an uncontrollable sugar addiction, and it makes you feel a horrible physical withdrawal when you try to remove sugar from your diet, Candida is a possible culprit. I have had patients who had severe Candida infections that caused them to be alcoholics. It's hard to know what comes first – the alcohol that causes the yeast to grow or the growth of the yeast after a course or two of antibiotics or a combination of all three. There is a phenomenon called auto-brewery syndrome in which a person can have fungal yeast form in the bowel that ferments ingested carbohydrates into alcohol. People with this condition become inebriated and suffer all the medical and social implications of alcoholism.

When you withdraw the yeast's food source – carbohydrates – they start dying off and release a toxin that makes you feel horrible. It's called a Herx reaction, which is short for Jarisch-Herxheimer's reaction. This toxin can cause brain fog, migraines, depression, anxiety, severe joint pain, and fatigue. What you need to do first is to get control of your body back. Sometimes, changing the diet is enough and sometimes you have to do more. Removing or reducing the food supply that feeds the yeast is just one layer.

Whatever it is, whether it is bacterial dysbiosis in the large intestine where there is an imbalance of the gut microbiome, yeast overgrowth, parasites, or worms, the next phase is to give an herbal antimicrobial or a combination of them. They differ from the conventional antibiotics in that they support the good bacteria and immune system and slowly remove the bad bacteria or bring the microbiome into proper balance.

Instead of dropping bombs and destroying everything in an area, we might instead send ground troops to manage things. We might even set up their army, build schools, homes, and roads. We use herbs to change the environment and make it unhabitable for the undesirable microbes and cultivate an environment for desirable microbes. Most pathogens only need a month supply of herbal antimicrobials, but Candida and other fungi can take three to twelve months.

Parasites and worms are easy to get rid of once they are found. They could potentially be a cause for the immune system not functioning because they actively turn off the immune system to escape detection. When that happens, as you can imagine, other problems ensue. Parasites have been around for ages. In the past, people would do cleanses twice a year with herbs. Some people think that a person gets parasites and worms only in third world countries, but they are in the US as well. They can be acquired walking on the beach or streams barefoot, swimming in lakes and rivers, eating lettuce bought at a farmer's market that hasn't been washed properly, and even in playground sandboxes. When I've found parasites or worms after testing and removed this layer with treatment, there is typically a reduction or remission of emotional, mental, and physical symptoms.

We can provide herbal antimicrobials based on symptoms alone or do a stool test. I use Diagnostic Solutions Lab's GIMAP (https://www.diagnosticsolutionslab.com/tests/gi-map) but there are other stool tests equally effective, like Genova Diagnostics GI Effects (https://www.gdx.net/product/gi-effects-comprehensive-stool-test). The stool test, unlike a conventional stool test, gives us a cross-section of what is happening in the colon in terms of bacterial, viral, fungal, parasitic, protozoa, and worms. It reports the imbalances and autoimmune triggers. It gives us information about the status of the immune response through obtaining secretory IgA levels and inflammation via calprotectin levels. It also tells me whether there is a problem with digesting fats and carbohydrates. We might give pancreatic enzymes to support digestion of carbohydrates and bile salts to assist with digesting fats.

When someone has a history of having to take antibiotics repeatedly for an infection, it usually means to me that they have biofilms. You know that slimy feeling on your shower curtain or that slimy feeling on the rocks when you cross a stream? Those are biofilms. Many microorganisms, after they colonize an area, build walls to protect themselves. A round of antibiotics in the bloodstream will kill the organisms outside of that film, but once the antibiotics are finished, survivors emerge from the biofilm and grow exponentially. This might cause another bout of infection *or* possibly a stalemate.

An example of this is a woman who has had recurrent UTI finds that she has a yeast infection and then takes an over-the-counter (OTC) antifungal for three to seven days. What she might be left with is a genital itch, urinary frequency, or urinary urgency. This is extremely common. I had an eight-year-old female patient who had been colonized with yeast. She would have to go to the bathroom every hour. Her teachers accused her of trying to get out of class and avoiding work. She was labeled with behavioral problems. Well, she really had to pee. The urinalysis was negative for bacterial infections, but they don't really test for fungal infections. She had urinary frequency from Candida. I would venture to say that most women under the age forty who have to wear incontinence underwear have fungal overgrowth, assuming that a structural abnormality has been ruled out. This is likely due to colonization of a pathogen in an area where it doesn't belong, or at a stalemate with the body's immune system, and/or protected by biofilms. I think some people's microbiome comes to a stalemate in some situations because they don't take the whole course of antibiotics as they should.

I recommend biofilm breakers through sources of food like garlic, onions, apple cider vinegar, pomegranates, and cinnamon. If that's not enough, I recommend herbs that break biofilms like oregano oil and turmeric or a supplement called Interfase from Klaire Labs or Kirkman Labs Biofilm Defense to break strong biofilms.

With yeast in particular, the toxins that are released cause a Herx reaction. I recommend activated charcoal thirty minutes after each dose of the antifungal, which binds the toxin to avoid this reaction. Because of the reaction, it sometimes takes months to get to the therapeutic dose. As I said, Candida is a bugger.

Clostridia difficile and Helicobacter pylori are two types of bacteria that are known pathogens. There are special ways of dealing with each. They are best left to investigate and handle with an experienced clinician. Clostridia difficile is well known for causing massive diarrhea after taking antibiotics. However it can also cause chronic infections that produce metabolites, 4-cresol, and HPHPA ((3-hydroxyphenyl)-3-hydroxypropionic acid) that inhibit dopamine beta hydroxylase, an enzyme that converts the neurotransmitter dopamine to norepinephrine. When this enzyme is inhibited, dopamine accumulates and can result in mental distress like schizophrenia, motor tics, or autism. Great Plains Laboratory's Organic Acid Test (OAT) is a urine test I frequently order to obtain these markers, yeast, and fungal markers. H. pylori is most associated with stomach ulcers or heartburn. However, on a chronic basis, it is associated with numerous conditions including depression and anxiety.

What I haven't mentioned is small intestinal bacterial overgrowth (SIBO). SIBO is an overgrowth of bacteria in the small intestine where it doesn't belong. This is a complicated condition that requires a special test called a hydrogen and methane breath test to detect it. This condition is one root cause of irritable bowel syndrome, which can cause a host of physical and emotional symptoms. There is extensive information about this condition that if you want to learn more, I recommend you go to Dr. Alison Siebecker's web resource: https://www.siboinfo.com/. She has made it her mission to provide a comprehensive guide to SIBO. I have had a number of patients with SIBO and once this was cleared up, the emotional symptoms cleared up as well.

Invisible hijackers are pathogenic microbes that take advantage of a weakened immune state setting off alarms alerting the immune system. For some people, one of those alarms is the symptom of depression. When the microbiome returns to homeostasis like a lush protected rain forest and it's being fed with what it needs to remain healthy, the rain barrel of inflammation is lowered and a layer is removed. After dietary changes, this layer effects the greatest change in symptom relief when done properly. There has been an explosion of research about the microbiome in the last five years, yet there is still much that we need to learn.

CHAPTER 9

Food Is Medicine and Food Is Poison

The F in SHIFT is for food. Your diet should provide a healthy balance of protein, carbs, and fat at each meal. The ultimate goal is to reduce inflammation. To do that, you will want to eat fewer inflammatory foods and more anti-inflammatory foods. Based on that premise, your diet ought to be filled with nutrient-dense foods that contain antioxidants devoid of processed foods. Antioxidants work by reducing levels of free radicals. These reactive molecules are created as a natural part of your metabolism but can lead to inflammation when there are too many.

There is no one perfect diet for a person. There are many books on the subject and people who tout a specific diet being great for them, but this same diet is denounced by another. I believe that diets ought to evolve over a person's lifespan, as everybody is different genetically, epigenetically, and everyone has different demands. The diet ought to evolve based on that individual's physiological demands and their own goals.

Understanding the geographic region where your ancestors came from gives you clues about how to change your health status for the future. If you remember, I told you about my mother and that she became quite ill with severe rheumatoid arthritis. As I mentioned earlier, I noticed as a teenager that when she was in India for several months most of her symptoms remitted. I thought it was because she was happy to be "home" but she corrected me and said her home was in the US. It was years later when I realized that it was the food that was different. Fresh vegetables and fruits, freshly caught seafood, curries, and rice (which are naturally gluten-free and cooked with fresh turmeric and healing spices), fresh milk from cows in nearby fields to make yogurt naturally overnight. If your family is from another country and was healthy while living there and then started to have health issues once they came to the US, it is possible that their body is rejecting the SAD (Standard American Diet). Go back to eating what you might in your "genetic homeland." Your genes want the food that they've known for thousands of years, not man-made processed foods. You inherit your microbiome while traveling through the birth canal. Your microbiome has evolved through generations of the maternal side of your family. In that evolution, it has become efficient in extracting nutrients, like iron, from vegetables in certain populations while other populations that subsist on meats have their iron readily available. Their microbiome doesn't have to work as hard. I believe this is why some people who come from generations of meat-eaters don't thrive as vegetarians. I've seen people cut out meat and thrive, and I've seen people eat meat and thrive.

I've seen people cut out gluten and dairy and all of their inflammatory symptoms drop significantly and others have found that soy was the issue for them. For my son, initially, it was all three, but he was able over the years to add some types of dairy back in. The key is to educate yourself about what types of problems are caused by which foods and see if these problems remit when you remove them. One way to know which foods to remove is to start with the ones you crave the most. Some people crave gluten (from wheat) and casein (from milk) because their bodies don't break down those proteins completely and make gliadorphin and casomorphin respectively. These are opioid peptides formed from incomplete digestion. If you must have that quart of ice cream every night or eat a bag of Goldfish regularly, think cravings and digestive issues. Some people can have intense withdrawal reactions similar to people with addictions because these morphine-like peptides bind to the μ receptor (or "mu receptor"), the same receptor for opiates. That's why some people get a "high" from eating dairy or gluten carbs and can't control their intake of these food groups. This is a clue about you that you need to note and it may be the first group of foods to pull out of the diet. There are reasons why people have strong cravings, and this, therefore requires further investigation.

I had a patient on the inpatient unit who was admitted because she was suicidal because she was in so much pain and her quality of life was non-existent. She didn't have a psychiatric problem per se, she was just sick and tired of being sick and tired. After getting a careful history of how things happened to her, she was able to tell me that she began to drink milk on a daily basis because her doctor told her to drink more fluids because she was dehydrated. She didn't like water. She chose milk. After a couple of years of this, she was drinking a full gallon of milk a day. As we were sitting there talking, her food tray was brought in and I asked her if she would be willing to do an experiment. I told her that food can be medicine and food can be poison and, given the timing of how things happened for her, I suspected that it was the milk and possibly other foods that could be causing her inflammation to her joints. While she was in the psychiatric unit, I proposed that she stop all dairy products during her stay and she said, "Sure, why not? I've got nothing to lose." And by the way, she agreed to drink water! She actually improved within forty-eight hours and most of her pain was gone by the time she was discharged.

Too much of something is usually not a good thing. I had a patient who was working out and intent on having a six-pack abdomen. He read somewhere that eating raw eggs every day was a good idea that he had a dozen raw eggs blended up daily. His symptoms improved rapidly just by stopping the eggs.

I use diets to shift physiology. While you are in consultation with me, I tailor the approach to your specific needs and base it on what you are capable of doing or willing to do that fits your lifestyle and capacity for energy. Some people chose to do food allergy (IgE) and food sensitivity (IgG) testing to determine which foods to pull out right away to affect a change. There are problems with food sensitivity testing in that there is a seventy-five to eighty percent rate of specificity and sensitivity because there is a lot of cross-reactivity between foods and the environment.

I believe that one needs to do their own personal investigations by doing what is called an elimination diet and, after at least twenty-one days without those foods (because twenty-one days is how long it takes to reduce IgG levels, the antibodies made in the body when sensitive to food). One can add one category back at a time and document any type of reaction. When it comes to symptoms that affect the brain, I prefer to have my patients remove gluten, dairy, and sugar for at least three months. If you notice a significant improvement within weeks of making this change, then the likelihood of having other significant causes is lower. If there is little to no change with eliminating foods on the elimination diet, that is a big clue to me that there are other layers to address - so we search for them. If you have a reaction to adding the foods back into the diet, then that category of food needs to stay out. The reasons why you have a reaction needs to be investigated so that at some point, the food or food group can be added back in. Sometimes, though, for some people, it might need to stay out long term to maintain homeostasis. This is why it's very important to keep a journal. Here are two possible scenarios: there might be increased gut impermeability, also known as leaky gut syndrome or you might not be digesting those foods properly – which then begs the question ...*why*?

With the advent of C-sections and people moving to all parts of the world, their microbiomes are subjected to different foods. Fortunately, according to the maternal microbiome legacy project, the practice of "vaginal seeding" has emerged, where a newborn delivered via Cesarean section is swabbed with the mother's vaginal secretions to transfer the mother's vaginal bacteria to the infant, mimicking what the infant would have been exposed to during vaginal birth. However, the benefits of "vaginal seeding" have not been evaluated and the safety of this practice has not been proven despite it coming into clinical use. A study is currently being conducted to determine if the maternal bacterial community is transferred to the infant during delivery and if the different types of deliveries alter this transfer. Having mother's milk, but especially the colostrum, the first milk, is important in establishing the immune system as well.

What's also important is not only the *type* of food eaten but the *source* of these foods. If the cow you eat has eaten inflammatory food, that will affect you, and if the vegetables you eat have been sprayed with pesticides, that will certainly affect you. When I was a kid, whenever I ate strawberries, my lips would tingle and swell a little and the strawberries were tart. I didn't really think I liked strawberries until I went to a farm where they grew them organically. We picked a bucket of them, but they didn't stay in the bucket long because they were so sweet and juicy. It was the first time I hadn't had any lip tingling. It was then that I realized it must be the pesticides that were sprayed on the strawberries that provoked my past reactions. It made me wonder if I was truly allergic to the food I thought I was allergic to or perhaps I was actually allergic to what was sprayed on them.

Annually, it's a good idea to go to www.ewg.org to get *The Dirty Dozen* and *The Clean 15* lists and go to https://www.nrdc.org/ for the *Mercury Guide* and *The Smart Seafood Buying Guide.* These organizations do not measure the level of contamination by glyphosate, more commonly known as Roundup, so eat organic as much as you are able.

There is much research that demonstrates that the Mediterranean diet is anti-inflammatory. Yes, a percentage of people did well. There are more strict variations of this diet like the modified Paleo diet, then the Paleo diet, then there is the Autoimmune Protocol (AIP) diet for autoimmune diseases. The Bulletproof diet and the Ketogenic diet are excellent for weight loss, insulin resistance, metabolic syndrome, and brain inflammation. I have had numerous patients whose depression, anxiety, and attention problems disappeared with the Ketogenic diet. Whole30 is a trendy but brilliant version of the elimination diet as well. And then there are vegetarian and veganism, the plant diets touted to be beneficial for heart disease and cancer. These are all healthy choices but only for some people. It is something to experiment with and see how you feel, but you should still listen to your body. Sometimes drastic changes can be hard if the demands of your body are high.

The differences in these diets are essentially the balance in amounts of protein, carbs, and fats. The goal is to take out the foods that cause inflammation for you and put in the foods that are healing for you.

Ultimately, all these diets eliminate all processed foods including sugar and unhealthy processed fats. If it's not made naturally, don't eat it. Return to eating real, whole foods made by the planet and not man. Most of these diets require a significant intake of a variety of vegetables and an increased intake of healthy fats. It's important to read all labels and rotate your foods every three days.

There are six major groups of food that most people are sensitive to and should try to remove – gluten, dairy, soy, corn, eggs, and nuts.

The elimination diet is too difficult for some people to do, but it is the "gold standard" for determining your food sensitivities. I find that many of my patients do not want to do the elimination diet but are willing to follow an anti-inflammatory diet. Inflammatory foods should be avoided for at least one month, but if you notice no difference, then extend it to three months as sometimes the inflammation takes longer to come down.

What to Eat for at Least One Month, but Ideally Three Months:

- Healthy carbs: quinoa and wild rice

- Vegetables: two-thirds of your plate. Eat as much as you want but don't overeat. Eat six to eight servings of vegetables – a rainbow of colors – a wide variety. Include options from the brassica family regularly (cabbage, cauliflower, Brussel sprouts, broccoli, broccoli sprouts, and kale). Sweet potatoes and yams are healthier choices compared to white potatoes. Eat veggies at every meal.

- Fruits: all berries, tart apples (Granny Smith), pomegranates, and cranberries. No other fruit is allowed.

- Healthy protein: meat and fish – six ounces of grass-fed beef, free-range chicken and turkey, grass-fed lamb, wild-caught fish and shellfish, organ meats, and wild game. Include them at every meal.

Healthy fats: coconut oil, coconut milk (full-fatted version only if canned or homemade), MCT oil (pure medium-chain triglycerides), extra virgin olive oil, olives, avocados, avocado oil, and lard from healthy animals. Cook only in oils that have high smoke points. You need fat in your diet to make hormones and to fuel the brain, as eighty percent of the brain is fat. Most people need more healthy fats, not less, in their diet. There is a very small percentage of people who should be on a low-fat diet. A cholesterol lower than 150 is associated with a heightened risk of developing major depressive disorder, as well as an increased risk of death from suicide.

- Fermented foods: sauerkraut, kimchi, real pickles. When I say real pickles, I mean the kind that are in the refrigerated section. They are raw, naturally fermented vegetables in a salty brine that produce live probiotics that are excellent for your gut. The pickles on the shelf made with vinegar do not contain live probiotics.

- Fluids: water, green tea, coconut kefir, water kefir (like Kevita), and bone broth. I find that water kefir is a great replacement for soda or alcohol.

- Sugar: Only stevia and monk fruit.

- If you are unsure about something and it's not on the list, don't eat it.

Avoid These Foods for One to Three Months:

- All processed foods: If it's packaged, don't eat it.

- Dairy: Avoid all animal milk products, including cheeses, yogurt, sour cream, whey protein, buttermilk, butter, ghee, kefir, ice cream, and cottage cheese.

- Avoid eggs.

- Grains (especially gluten): No wheat, rye, barley, corn, oats, kamut, sorghum, spelt, teff, or white rice.

- Nightshade vegetables: Avoid all white potatoes, tomatoes and tomato products, eggplant, sweet bell peppers (all colors), hot peppers, and cayenne pepper. Note: sweet potatoes and yams are fine to eat.

- Fruit: Avoid all fruit with high sugar content.

- Unhealthy meat and fish: Avoid grain/corn-fed or corn-"finished" beef, commercial chicken, turkey, pork and lamb, farm-raised fish and shellfish, organ meat from unhealthy animals, large predator fish that are high in mercury (mackerel, bluefish, albacore tuna, swordfish, and shark).

- Unhealthy fats: Avoid all trans or hydrogenated fat (found in processed or prepackaged foods), rancid fats (smells like turpentine), and vegetable oils other than those listed above in foods you can eat.

- Nuts: Avoid all nuts and nut-derived oils. This includes almonds, walnuts, cashews, pecans, Brazil nuts, pine nuts, hazelnuts and pistachios, including all nut oils, flours, and butter.

- Seeds: Avoid all seeds, such as pumpkin seeds, sesame seeds, flaxseed, chia seed, hemp seed, poppy seed, sunflower seeds, including all seed oils, flours, and butter.

- Beans and legumes: Avoid all beans (black, kidney, black-eyed peas, garbanzo, fava, white beans, lentils, and split peas) and legumes (soy, peanuts, and green beans).

- Sugar: Avoid all sugars added to food as well as high sugar content foods such as most fruits. This includes agave, honey, cane sugar, rice syrup, maple syrup, barley malt, corn syrup, molasses, and turbinado sugar.

- Artificial sweeteners: Avoid all sugar substitutes and artificial sweeteners including sucralose, Splenda, fake stevia, aspartame, and sugar alcohols (such as mannitol, sorbitol, dextrose, and xylitol).

- Avoid coffee, tea, soda, and alcohol.

After one to three months, reintroduce only one new food at a time. Eat it two to three times in the same day, stop eating it, then wait a full seventy-two hours to see if you have a reaction. Assess your response over that time, keeping track of your symptoms below. If there is no reaction to a food, you can keep that food in your food plan and continue with the next food for reintroduction. If you are unsure whether you had a reaction, retest the same food in the same manner. If you require more space, copy the blank chart for a second page.

	Day 1	Day 2	Day 3	Day 4
Time:				
Food:				
Digestion/ Bowel Function:				
Joint/ Muscle Aches:				
Headache/ Pressure:				
Nasal or Chest Congestion:				
Kidney/Bladder Function:				
Skin:				
Energy Level:				
Sleep:				
Other Symptoms:				

Gluten and dairy ought to be the last food groups you add. Nowadays everyone reacts to gluten on some level. There is a great deal of dispute over this particular class, and the only way to know is to add it back in and see.

However, there is one caveat to this plan. If you notice no improvement in your symptoms in one month, then stay on the diet for another month. The best way to know that you are improving is to do the MSQ again and see if the total drops. Don't rely just on how you feel because how you feel emotionally will color your judgment. People are often surprised when they compare the MSQ score at the beginning and when they repeat the questionnaire. Some people deem the diet a failure, meaning a lack of change in symptoms, and then start adding foods back in too soon. My interpretation is that it is one layer that has been removed and its proof that there are definitely other layers to go after. Now we need to find and remove the other layers. Also, you will learn about the repair phase of the Five Rs in chapter 12. Ideally, you will want to repair the gut lining before you add foods back into your diet. When the gut lining is healed, you will likely tolerate the reintroduction of foods better.

Wheat, which is a major source of gluten, has been changed over the past fifty years with the advent of hybridizing to make it drought- and disease-resistant, processing it differently, and then adding it into everything we eat just so it gives foods like condiments that velvety texture. These have dramatically increased the concentration of glutenin and gliadin in our food.

It takes a long time to reintroduce foods and wait for a possible reaction. It takes diligence and time. If you accidentally eat something that is not on the diet, don't beat yourself up, just be curious and notice if there is any reaction or change. Ultimately, the body tells you what it needs and wants for healing. So *you* need to listen.

I find that the hardest part of the day is breakfast. Firstly, there is no law saying you can't have lunch or dinner at breakfast time. Secondly, there are things that are delicious that you likely haven't tried. You can have golden milled flax meal, white chia seeds, or amaranth with cinnamon and coconut milk and it's better than oatmeal. A green smoothie with or without a protein powder is easy to make and there are thousands of recipes online. Almond flour is a great substitute for recipes and cassava flour is a winner as it is the closest one to gluten in how it binds and prevents crumbling.

When you go shopping, start reading the labels on the back of the products instead of the front of the product and chose products that have fewer and real ingredients that you can read, pronounce, and recognize. Avoid the aisles in the middle of the store as the most processed foods are shelf-stable and don't require refrigeration. If it doesn't spoil or grow, it's fake food. Know what you are putting on or in your body or in your air. As you run out of products, replace them with "cleaner" products. It's not necessary to do a complete overhaul, but if you're one of those people who likes a fresh start, then be my guest.

I have one warning about doing an elimination or anti-inflammatory diet. If you have any type of disordered eating, restricting foods can trigger an eating disorder. I recommend that you work with a functional nutritionist to help you through this process.

I hope you can see that food is medicine for some and poison for others. The trick is figuring out which foods are healing for you and harmful to you. Food provides energy, nutrients, and runs lines of communication on a cellular level. It represents love, connection, and is nurturing in more ways than one. Depriving oneself from food alone can lead to suffering in many ways, depression being one of them. It's more than calories in and calories out; it's a way of life.

CHAPTER 10

Stress - Know Your Triggers

"When the sunshine of loving kindness
meets the tears of suffering, the
rainbow of compassion arises."
– A meditation teacher from Myanmar

Stress is the S in SHIFT.

One actually needs a healthy amount of stress to keep the immune system in shape. I talked about the role of inflammation in the body, which can cause oxidative stress to the body. Not providing the body what it needs can cause a significant amount of stress. We take our bodies for granted and ignore these signs, believing that it's all part of "normal." Having no bowel movement for a week is not normal, menstrual cramps are not normal, menopause should not be painful and uncomfortable, and needing coffee to wake up is not normal. These problems are caused by stress but are also stressful to the body. There are normal transitions in life that can also be stressful periods to our body and if other stressors are present at the same time, the body goes tilt. Those periods are puberty, all the different stages of pregnancy, and menopause.

A normal response to stress is typically a rush of adrenalin that increases your heart rate, dilates your blood vessels getting the blood flowing to your brain, lungs, and muscles, dilates your eyes so you can see danger, and dumps glucose in the bloodstream to provide these organs energy. Everything else in the body slows or shuts down to conserve energy. This is your sympathetic nervous system in action to save your life from a perceived danger. Once the danger is over, cortisol is released to shut off the adrenalin and then the system returns to normal. However, if that stress occurs repeatedly, then adrenalin remains chronically high and then cortisol also remains chronically high.

Adrenalin and cortisol can cause chronic physiological changes in the brain and body that appear to be other illnesses but are just an extreme reaction to stress. Hypertension is a well-known example. Less well-known examples are elevated blood sugars and cholesterol, which are more commonly associated with diabetes and heart disease. Stress alone can raise these markers.

If this begins early in childhood during a time when the body, brain, immune system, and hormonal system are developing, the wear and tear start before the child has had a chance to mature enough to handle it. To determine how much impact stress has on a person during childhood, I have patients complete an ACE questionnaire. You may have already completed this when I linked it in Chapter 6, but if not, I recommend doing it now: https://www.acesconnection.com/blog/got-your-ace-resilience-scores.

The ACE or Adverse Childhood Experiences Study was conducted by Dr. Vince Felitti at Kaiser Permanente and Dr. Bob Anda at the Center for Disease Control. Between 1995 and 1997, they asked seventeen thousand, five hundred adults about their history of exposure to what they called "adverse childhood experiences," or ACEs. Those include physical, emotional, or sexual abuse; physical or emotional neglect; a family member with mental illness, substance dependence, incarceration; loss of a parent through separation, divorce or other reason; or domestic violence. For every question answered "yes", you would get a point on your ACE score. About half of the participants were male; seventy-five percent were Caucasian; the average age was fifty-seven; seventy five percent had attended college; all had jobs and good health care.

The researchers correlated these ACE scores against health outcomes after following them for years. What they discovered was that ACEs are incredibly common. Sixty-four percent of the population had at least one ACE, and one in eight had four or more ACEs. They also learned that there was a dose-response relationship between ACEs and health outcomes: the higher your ACE score, the worse your health outcomes. For a person with an ACE score of four or more, their relative risk of depression was four point five times. For suicidality, it was twelve times. People with an ACE score of four are twice as likely to be smokers and seven times more likely to be an alcoholic. However, it doesn't affect just one's mental health or behavior alone. A person with an ACE score of seven or more had three times the lifetime risk of lung cancer and three point five times the risk of ischemic heart disease, the number one killer in the United States of America. People with an ACE score of six or higher are at risk of their lifespan being shortened by twenty years. The ACE questionnaire is not perfect. Since the publishing of the ACE questionnaire, there have been revisions over the years to include other types of trauma as well as a Resilience Questionnaire.

Your thinking might be that if you've had a difficult childhood, you're more likely to drink, smoke, and do all these things that are going to ruin your health. Believe or not, even if you don't engage in any high-risk behavior, you're still more likely to develop heart disease or cancer. The reason for this has to do with the hypothalamic-pituitary-adrenal axis, the brain's and body's stress response system, called the autonomic nervous system that controls our fight-flight-freeze response – the sympathetic drive and our rest and digest response – the parasympathetic drive. Your parasympathetic system is what kicks in to bring you back to baseline as the body prefers to be in homeostasis. It is in this state that one is at rest and is able to digest. In fact, some people are unable to digest their food because they are in a chronic state of fight-flight-freeze. As a result, some people become deficient in certain vitamins and minerals. Chronic stimulation of the sympathetic drive can also cause increased gut permeability and suppression of your immune system.

Stimulating the vagus nerve supports the parasympathetic system. Gargling, humming, and taking cold showers are all techniques to lower your stress level. I had a patient notice that her Raynaud's (numbness and pain due to reduced blood flow) in her fingertips improved. Another patient had a signif-icant improvement in his depression with exercise followed by cold showers, worsening of symptoms when stopped, and improvement when started again.

As you can see, stress alone can start a cascade of mental and physical symptoms through a variety of physiological mechanisms. Knowing your ACE score helps us to know how early that stress began and consequently how low your thresh-old is for stress. Stress from trauma can appear in the body before you are cognitively aware of it in your mind. The body keeps the score.

Furthermore, when cortisol levels remain elevated chronically, it affects other hormones. This is where the H in SHIFT comes in. When stress levels are high, the cortisol is a response to adrenalin like a runaway train. If the body doesn't respond to cortisol, the body puts on the break, or downregulates the thyroid to bring the body into homeostasis. There is an explosion of hypothyroidism in this country. My belief is that some of what seems like hypothyroidism is truly the body's response to stress. The body slows everything down as a way to force it to rest. Our bodies are very intelligent! However, there are many other reasons why the thyroid may not be functioning efficiently. Hypothyroidism is a common cause of depression. There is great disagreement between conventional doctors and functional medicine doctors about how to test and even how to interpret thyroid testing. Conventional doctors might only look at one lab test, the TSH (thyroid-stimulating hormone). They might believe that if the TSH is normal, then the entire feedback loop of communication between the hypothalamus (that releases TRH - thyrotropin-releasing hormone - to stimulate the pituitary gland in the brain) to release TSH that regulates the production of thyroid hormone – is normal – because the feedback loop supposedly would feed back a problem. Functional medicine doctors test the entire loop where they are able, by ordering the TSH, free T3, free T4 and reverse T3. Some even order the total T3 and total T4. There are numerous nutrients that the thyroid needs to convert the inactive form of T4 to the active form, T3.

Conventional doctors don't typically test for cortisol level unless they are looking for a specific disease process: abnormally high cortisol called Cushing's disease or abnormally low cortisol called Addison's disease. They might do a serum cortisol test in the morning. Functional medicine practitioners are more concerned about everyday functioning, the rhythms, and how these rhythms impact other rhythms in the body. They might do a salivary cortisol test that is collected four times throughout the day. I believe that doctors ought to be concerned about both the serum cortisol and the salivary cortisol levels in the same way that a police officer might be concerned about a car weaving on a road differently than a car that's left the road and crashed. Do you get my drift?

Furthermore, there is a phenomenon called "pregnenolone steal" that converts all of the sex hormones into cortisol because in times of stress, it is more important to survive than to make babies. There are many studies that show that stress is one of many reasons why the infertility rates are high in this country. Having an imbalance of estrogen, progesterone, and testosterone can certainly impact your mood among other things.

We discussed the role of sleep and exercise in reducing inflammation in the body. These also reduce stress in the body. There are other things you can do as well, but they require investing time to build a daily practice. There is much research that demonstrates that deep breathing, mindfulness meditation, and yoga reduce stress by supporting the parasympathetic system – the rest and digest system. Finding a practice that fits your personality and lifestyle is important.

In college, I learned about supporting the parasympathetic system by eliciting the *Relaxation Response,* written about by Herbert Benson, M.D. in 1975. This concept has been around for a long time. It's a wonder that every single doctor in the country doesn't demand that their patients practice it. It's a Westernized form of transcendental meditation that was validated by research. It's a seven-step process that relaxes the body. Here are the steps:

1. Sit quietly in a comfortable position.

2. Close your eyes.

3. Deeply relax all your muscles, beginning at your feet and progressing up to your face. Keep them relaxed. [Relax your tongue – and thoughts will cease.]

4. Breathe through your nose. Become aware of your breathing. As you breathe out, say the word "one"* silently to yourself. For example, breathe in, and then out, and say "one,"* in and out, and repeat "one."* Breathe easily and naturally.

5. Continue for ten to twenty minutes. You may open your eyes to check the time, but do not use an alarm. When you finish, sit quietly for several minutes, at first with your eyes closed and later with your eyes opened. Do not stand up for a few minutes.

6. Do not worry about whether you are successful in achieving a deep level of relaxation. Maintain a passive attitude and permit relaxation to occur at its own pace. When distracting thoughts occur, try to ignore them by not dwelling upon them and return to repeating "one."*

7. With practice, the response should come with little effort. Practice the technique once or twice daily, but not within two hours after any meal, since the digestive processes seem to interfere with the elicitation of the Relaxation Response.
   *Choose any soothing, mellifluous-sounding word, preferably with no meaning or association, to avoid stimulation of unnecessary thoughts.

Deep breathing is something that can be done by anyone, anywhere, and at any time. You can learn many different types of breathing patterns. I typically recommend starting this simple one. Breathe in through your nose, hold the breath for a few seconds, and then exhale through your mouth. The time it takes to exhale should be about twice what it is to inhale. I suggest a 4:2:7 pattern – 4 to inhale, 2 to hold, and 7 to exhale. Let go of other thoughts while you breathe. You might consider inhaling a color (blue) and exhaling a different color (red) or breathing in a word (love) and exhaling another word (hate). You choose whatever feels right to you - your own colors or words.

There are several apps you can download onto your smart phone or iPad. Some popular ones are Calm, Insight Timer, Headspace, and Aura. This is the easiest and fastest way to start a practice if you are a beginner. The Wim Hof Method is a combination of breathing exercises and meditation while gradually exposing yourself to cold shower therapy.

Jon Kabat-Zinn, Ph. D., is best known for his teachings in mindfulness meditation. A guided mindfulness meditation series and others are on his YouTube channel: https://www.youtube.com/watch?v=8HYLyuJZKno&feature=share.

One of my favorite guided meditations is Omvana – 6 Phase Guided Meditation by Vishen Lakhiani: https://www.youtube.com/watch?v=EaRu14P9H84.

There are a few practices that aren't as well known that have helped a number of my patients. One is called the Emotional Freedom Technique (EFT), which is also known as tapping. Here is an introductory video to tapping: https://youtu.be/pAclBdj2oZU.

A popular site for tapping is Tapping Solutions (https://www.thetappingsolution.com/tapping-101/) created by Nick and Jessica Ortner.

HeartMath (https://www.heartmath.com/) is a powerful way to modulate stress quickly. You can order the Inner Balance app for your phone or buy the instrument separately. The website describes how it changes your heart rhythm pattern to create physiological coherence; a scientifically measurable state characterized by increased order and harmony in our mind, emotions, and body. It essentially teaches you how to turn on your parasympathetic nervous system through biofeedback. Dynamic Neural Training System (https://retrainingthebrain.com) is a program that would help retrain your limbic system, but you need to dedicate four days to do the training followed by one hour a day for six months.

Option B (https://optionb.org) helps people build resilience and find meaning in the face of adversity.

Recently a patient also informed me of an app called Ten Percent Happier (https://www.tenpercent.com/) that teaches meditation and other courses.

These are some practices I've introduced to help calm down the body. There is a saying, "If it's worth doing, it's worth doing right." The only way to know which feels right for you is to try it, but if you're going to try it, it has to be done wholeheartedly. I suggest you pick one and do it wholeheartedly for two weeks and see how you feel.

Sometimes the mind is whirling like a tornado and people don't even realize that the mind is creating an intense amount of stress. If you've lived your life this way, you may not have a frame of reference of what normal is. How would you know? Your perceptions of the world are influenced by your parents and your reactions are modeled by your parents. Stress is determined by your perceptions of the world and your ability to respond to it. Temperament, faith, desire, and courage bolster your ability to respond. I tell my patients that life is like the weather. Learning to look at the weather report and preparing for it is the best you can do. If you get caught in a rainstorm or a nor'easter, you need to know how to respond. Having the ability to act reduces depression and feeling confident in the response reduces anxiety. Actively surveying where you feel trapped, stuck, or helpless in situations are clues to sources of stress that result in both anxiety and depression. This reflects stress related to yourself interacting with the world *outside* of you.

You could also have stress related to yourself interacting with the world *inside* of you. Some people have automatic negative thoughts or cognitive distortions. Many of these thoughts are a product of habit. They remain strong because of the power of belief. Once you stop believing certain things about yourself or the world, it's just a matter of removing the habit of it being in your mind. Some people are ruled by feelings of guilt, shame, anger, and fear that get in the way of what they want in life. I tell my patients: "Never make any decisions based on shame, fear, guilt, or anger. Do it because you choose to do it." Then contend with these emotions separately as they generally arise from some past trauma or conflict. These issues respond well to psychotherapy. The key to success in psychotherapy is to have self-compassion and connection.

"Stress" is a general term that means something different to everybody. Stress can be motivating, yet also destructive. It can toughen you up or cause you to crumble. Ultimately, stress will always be a part of life. Learning to recognize where the stress resides, whether it be emotional, physical, or spiritual, and determining how to respond is a skill that needs to be mastered. This requires patience, empathy, curiosity, and kindness. Much of what I've discussed in this chapter might not be new to you. The most important piece is that stress can impact the gut, causing increased gut permeability.

CHAPTER 11

Toxic Burden

I'm dating myself here, but do you remember the movie *The Boy in the Plastic Bubble*? The main character had to live a bubble because he had no immune system. Thankfully, scientists were able to create a toxin barrier for him.

Guess what? You already have a barrier, and it is working every single moment whether you are awake or asleep. That barrier is your microbiome, which is an army that makes up your immune system. It keeps toxins out and keeps you safe from the assault on your body on a daily basis. You don't even know it until the barrier is breached.

The most obvious toxins are cigarettes and alcohol. If you haven't quit smoking, that's a no brainer. By now, you're making a fully informed choice to harm yourself. That's your right. But think about the overall effect on your mind and body. Is it worth it? Cigarette smoking doesn't just affect your lungs. It affects your entire body. Alcohol is a big part of our culture and affects people differently. People think that they have to be an alcoholic for alcohol to affect their health, but any alcohol consumption can affect the gut lining significantly. Alcohol is a toxin! It acts like turpentine to the gut lining and it is worth stopping alcohol for at least eight weeks to allow the microvilli to grow back. When you are having mental and physical symptoms that are causing you distress, it helps to remove all possible toxins including cigarettes and alcohol despite these being legal.

When people think of toxic exposure, they think about lead or other heavy metals. Most people have heard of lead poisoning in children due to lead paint. Laws have been passed to protect our children. However, there are other metals that are concerning like mercury in fish (that for some reason only pregnant women are alerted to avoid) and arsenic in pressure-treated wood. Government regulations permit small levels to be present in the belief that our bodies can and will appropriately detox them out. They even let our Vitamin B12 be made as cyano-cobalamin. That's one cyanide molecule that is attached to cobalamin – another name for Vitamin B12. The body then has to expend energy to remove the cyanide molecule from the body. There are other forms of Vitamin B12 that are safer and frankly easier for our bodies to use, but the cyanocobalamin is "shelf-stable," allowing it to remain on the shelf without spoiling. What authorities don't yet acknowledge is that the cumulative effect of all of the toxins around us at some point overwhelm our immune system. Again, I might be dating myself, but what comes to mind is the episode of *I Love Lucy* where Lucy has the job of wrapping up chocolates that are going by on a conveyor belt. She starts off thinking it's easy but then the conveyor belt goes faster and faster and she can't keep up.

Think about your exposure to toxins. My husband recalls running through a campsite behind a truck spraying pesticides because it was cool. I remember as a child the small airplane above me spraying the trees as they had an infestation of tent caterpillars. And what about your neighbors' perfect lawn, in which you ran barefoot and absorbed the pesticides keeping it that way.

There are certain jobs that have chronic exposure to chemicals such as hair stylists, manicurists, makeup artists, painters, welders, cleaners, auto mechanics, highway and airport workers, and golf course workers and players.

There are thousands of new chemicals produced every year, and we have no idea if they are safe for us. The US government does not practice the precautionary principle, but our European friends do. The principle implies that there is a social responsibility to protect the public from exposure to harm when scientific investigation has found a plausible risk. These protections can be relaxed only if further scientific findings emerge that provide sound evidence that no harm will result. Instead, it seems that the US government puts the burden on people to prove that harm was done by a chemical exposure.

Some conventional doctors believe that toxins are only a concern if they're in the bloodstream. Getting serum blood levels is easy for known toxins. But what about the unknown toxins? Aside from that, very few doctors ask about toxin exposure. Functional medicine practitioners are concerned about the body burden and how much is sitting in our organs mucking up their ability to function efficiently, our exposure from all angles – through our skin, our lungs, and in everything that we put in our mouth. There is a nonprofit professional medical society that aims to raise awareness of the environmental causes of inflammatory illnesses and to support the recovery of individuals affected by these illnesses through the integration of clinical practice, education, and research: https://iseai.org.

We need to listen to what our body is telling us when it smells. Body odor is not normal to have. It's a sign that something is off in your gut and liver that you aren't eliminating very well, and toxins are coming out of your body through your skin and producing an odor. It's normal to have some odor in the course of the day, which should improve with a shower, and it's normal to have some odor after exerting yourself, but a heavy odor all day long is concerning. There are different types of smells. It's typically caused by certain foods that your body doesn't like. Rather than asking *why*, we think it's just normal and cover it up with perfume or deodorant – chemicals that your immune system then has to flush out.

We have been putting creams, makeup, sunscreen, and mosquito repellent on our skin and using hair care products that are full of synthetic toxins. These toxins get into our bloodstream and make our bodies work hard to eliminate them. Research has shown that triclosan, the hand sanitizer, is a big culprit for destroying our immune system. The best way to sanitize our hands is with plain soap and water.

We are using all sorts of cleansers for our homes, synthetic air fresheners, and pesticides. If you must scent the air, try to find natural alternatives like aromatherapy with real, not synthetic, essential oils. Soap and water go a long way. Bleach is not the best thing, especially for mold, as it can potentially cause the release of mold toxins, depending on the type of mold, and make things worse.

Conventional doctors often don't believe in detoxification. This word connotes multiple meanings. To me, it's about maximizing the efficacy of the current systems that filter out toxins – the liver, kidneys, colon, and lungs. Conventional doctors are taught that our organs function fine until they don't and that there is not much you can do about it when that happens. These filtering systems can get overwhelmed in the same way an air filter in a car can get overwhelmed in a dust storm. You might get a new filter for the car, but you can't do that with the body. Detoxing is providing the body nutrients to help these systems work more efficiently and providing herbs to clear out the muck left behind.

Think about your exposures and add them to your timeline you created in Chapter 6.

I had a friend who was getting severe reactions on her skin. She worked with a functional medicine doctor and it took a while to figure out that it was being caused by the chemicals on her clothes from the dry cleaners. She had to get rid of all of her clothes, but she regained her health. Yes, there are organic dry-cleaning companies.

Here is an Environmental Toxin Questionnaire to jog your memory and get an overview for yourself. This questionnaire is meant to get you thinking about your current and past exposure. If you find that you have had some current exposures, do what you can to eliminate the sources. If there are past exposures, I recommend that you discuss your findings with someone knowledgeable about these things and obtain advice about how to address them.

FOOD & WATER	Yes	Sometimes	In the Past	No
1. Do you consume conventionally-farmed (non-organic) or genetically-modified fruits and vegetables?				
2. Do you consume conventionally-raised (non-organic) animal products (i.e., meat, poultry, dairy, eggs)?				
3. Do you consume canned or farmed fish and seafood?				
4. Do you consume processed foods (i.e., foods with added artificial colors, flavors, preservatives, or sweeteners), deep-fried, or fast foods?				
5. Do you drink water from a well, spring, or cistern, or from plumbing pipes or fixtures installed before 1986?				
6. Do you drink sodas, juices, or other beverages with natural or refined sweeteners (i.e., high-fructose corn syrup, cane sugar, agave nectar, Stevia, undiluted fruit juice, etc.) or artificial sweeteners (i.e., NutraSweet/Equal/aspartame, Sweet'N Low/saccharine, Splenda/sucralose, Sunett/Sweet One/acesulfame K, neotame)?				

HOME & WORK ENVIRONMENT	Yes	Sometimes	In the Past	No
1. Do you live in an apartment or home built before 1978, or in a mobile home, boat, or RV?				
2. Does your home or workplace contain new construction materials or furniture (i.e., paint, laminate flooring, particle board, new carpeting, bedding, furniture, etc.)?				
3. Does your home or workplace show signs of mold or water damage (i.e., cracking paint, ceiling leaks, decaying insulation or foam, visible mold, or damp windows, basement, or crawlspaces, etc.)?				
4. Are you exposed to toxic substances (i.e., treated lumber, lead paint, paint chips or dust, broken mercury thermometers or fluorescent bulbs, etc.) at home or work?				
5. Are you exposed to conventional cleaning chemicals, disinfectants, hand sanitizers, air fresheners, scented candles, or other scented products at home or work?				
6. Do you live or work near an industrial pollution source (i.e., highway, factory, incinerator, gas station, power plant, etc.)?				

	Yes	Sometimes	In the Past	No
7. Do you live or work near a source of electromagnetic radiation (i.e., cell phone tower, high-voltage power lines, or other known source)?				
8. Do you live or work in an agricultural area or another type of area where you are exposed to herbicides, pesticides, or fungicides?				
9. Do you have wood-burning, propane, or gas stoves or appliances at home or work?				
10. Do you live or work in a sealed building with recirculated air?				
TRAVEL & RECREATION				
1. Do you frequent parks, golf courses, or other outdoor or recreational areas treated with herbicides, pesticides, or fungicides?				
2. Do you travel by air?				
3. Do you run or bike to work along busy streets?				
4. Do you get sick while camping, hiking, or traveling (foreign or domestic)?				
5. Are you exposed to toxic chemicals as a result of a hobby (i.e., paints, photo-developing chemicals, epoxy adhesives, glues, varnishes, etc.)?				

MEDICAL & PERSONAL CARE	Yes	Sometimes	In the Past	No
1. Are you sensitive to personal care products like lotions, moisturizers, toners, shampoos, conditioners, shaving creams, and soaps?				
2. Are you sensitive to smoke, perfumes, fragrances, cleaning products, gasoline, or other fumes?				
3. Do you smoke, or are you often exposed to second-hand smoke?				
4. Do you have a history of heavy use of alcohol, or recreational or prescription drugs?				
5. Do you have any unusual reactions to anesthesia or to prescription or over-the-counter medications?				
6. Do you have root canals, extracted teeth, "silver" fillings, crowns, dental sealants, dentures, retainers, aligning trays, braces, mouth guards, dental implants, etc.?				
7. Do you have food reactions, sensitivities, or intolerances? Do you have environmental allergies?				
8. Do you have any artificial materials in your body (implants, pins, joints, etc.)?				
9. Do you lead a high-stress lifestyle, or have you experienced a stressful or traumatic event?				

Note: Used with permission from The Institute for Functional Medicine (IFM), the global leader in Functional Medicine and a collaborator in the transformation of healthcare. IFM is a 501(c)(3) nonprofit organization that believes Functional Medicine can help every individual reach their full potential for health and well-being. Under no circumstances may the whole or any part of the materials be translated into another language, nor may you create derivative or other works without IFM's prior written permission (for permission please contact info@ifm.org).

Here is a free survey to quickly screen yourself: https://www. lhscience.com/toxicity-survey.

Do a survey of your environment and all of the products you use. Are they all really necessary? Ultimately, we want to find a balance between our environment and our immune system and use products wisely while looking for healthier alternatives. We can choose to limit our exposure to toxins by becoming more aware of our surroundings and what we choose to put in or on our bodies.

There is a list of foods on the Environmental Working Group website that tells you which foods are safe to buy that are not organic and which to buy that are organic. The website for The Natural Resources Defense Council (https://www.nrdc. org/stories/smart-seafood-buying-guide) can give you a list of the types of seafood that are safest. These lists are updated annually. Another website called Skin Deep (https://www.ewg. org/skindeep/) allows you to put your makeup brand into a search tool to inform you of what toxins are in it.

One class of toxins that I want to mention is called endocrine disruptors. Endocrine disruptors can mimic or partly mimic naturally occurring hormones in the body like estrogens (the female sex hormone), androgens (the male sex hormone), and thyroid hormones, potentially producing overstimulation, and bind to a receptor within a cell and block the endogenous hormone from binding to it resulting in an under-stimulation. Either way, it results in a hormone imbalance. These chemicals can make someone feel like they are going into early menopause, cause men to have man boobs, and cause weight gain. By the way, it's not normal to have man boobs and it's not due to weight gain. Hormonal changes have the same root cause for both the weight and man boobs, formally known as gynecomastia.

Many people have become aware of the BPA, or bisphenol A, in plastic bottles. Everyone threw them out and bought BPA-free plastic bottles. Guess what? These bottles are BPA-free but not free of a different kind of bisphenol, bisphenol S and bisphenol F, which are just as bad. Plastic items labeled with the recycling numbers 3 and 7 or the letters "PC" likely contain BPA, BPS, or BPF. Fortunately, people are catching on. The safest bottles are glass and stainless steel. There are many products that contain BPA: like thermal printer register receipts, feminine hygiene products, and canned foods. There are other types of estrogen disruptors as well. You can get a list of the Dirty Dozen Endocrine Disruptors on the Environmental Working Group website. They offer alternative products that are EWG-verified as being safe. To avoid plastic in your food, try not to heat food or liquids in plastic or pouches. High heat allows the plastic to leech chemicals faster. Don't drink coffee in Styrofoam cups or take-home food in Styrofoam containers. Again, restaurants are catching on to these toxin exposures. If you have a favorite restaurant, ask them to switch to paper containers and paper cups.

There was a time when I was using a lot of makeup and hair products. I had my nails done every other week with acrylic nails. I had severe eczema requiring multiple creams and wore perfumes and deodorants. I stopped all of it during my health journey and returned to a few products that I knew weren't affecting me. I did return to using dishwasher pods and laundry soap, but I am much more mindful of what I buy.

Once toxins come into our bodies, they may accumulate and cause inflammation. We can support our bodies by eating the right foods and reducing stress to the body in other ways as discussed in previous chapters. You can boost your immune system by helping it work more efficiently with vitamins and minerals and possibly doing an annual liver cleanse. There are supplements that you can take if you are aware of a specific exposure, but in this case, it would be best to work with someone to complete a thorough assessment and make recommendations.

The body is a beautiful machine that has the capacity to adapt to the environment but only up to a point. Toxins accumulate over time and overwhelm the immune system, resulting in inflammation, and possibly contributing to depression. Every year there are new toxic chemicals added to the environment that our bodies don't even recognize. I hope someday we might be able to change policy regarding regulation of exposure of new innovations to the public at large. In the meantime, we have the power to help ourselves by increasing our awareness, limiting our exposure, and fueling our bodies to eliminate these toxins efficiently.

CHAPTER 12

Shore Up Your Defenses

We talked about *Removing* causes of inflammation – inflammatory foods, infections, toxins and stress – and *Replacing* with nutrients and foods that reduce inflammation. Those are the first two Rs – remove and replace. Because of poor choices in food or problems with digesting, some people have been depleted for so long that their wells are dry, therefore taking a highly absorbable multivitamin with minerals and phytonutrients helps to replace what's missing while getting a food plan established.

Once we've removed the unhealthy foods and replaced them with healthy foods and nutrients, removed the chronic infections and removed toxins from the body and the environment, we want to replace unhealthy habits with healthy habits to reduce stress.

The next R is *Re-inoculating* the gut microbiome with probiotics.

The healthy gut is home to trillions of bacteria and the type and diversity of bacteria have a major influence on our mental and physical health and influence our behavior and personality. Just like other ecosystems, like the rainforest or an aquarium, some species have positive effects on our health while others are harmful pathogens. It is the balance that keeps each of them in check. There are some bacteria that are usually harmless but can become harmful if left unchecked.

Probiotics are used to improve your immune system by restoring and maintaining order and to populate the gut micro-biome while crowding out and preventing unwelcome bacteria and other pathogens from colonizing.

The best way to get probiotics into your gut is through your diet. Eating fermented foods at every meal is ideal. Most Asian cultures include fermented foods on every plate, like pickled ginger on a Japanese dish or mango pickle with an Indian dish followed by yogurt at the end of the meal. This is not common in the US. The closest thing would be a pickled cucumber accompanying chips and a sandwich. Sauerkraut, other pickled vegetables, kimchi, different types of yogurt, and miso are other options. Nowadays, there are cultured beverages readily available like kombucha and kefir – dairy, water, or coconut. There is a growing trend to understand the importance of probiotics in parts of the US.

Certain foods in our diets nourish the gut bacteria and help them to multiply and thrive. The foods that nourish the probiotic bacteria are called prebiotics. Prebiotics are carbohydrates that may largely be indigestible for us, but our gut bacteria can digest them. So, including these dietary carbohydrates helps to increase the numbers of beneficial bacteria.

Here is a list of some foods and herbs that contain the prebiotic inulin, an oligosaccharide that is a type of complex carbohydrate that feeds gut bacteria: asparagus, apples, beans, burdock root, chicory root, cocoa, dandelion root and greens, flax seeds, garlic, green bananas, Jerusalem artichokes, jicama root, leeks, oats, onions, and plantains.

When fed, your gut bacteria produce short-chain fatty acids, such as butyrate, acetate, and propionate. These acids lower the pH of the colon, which prevents the growth of pathogens. Short-chain fatty acids also provide food for the cells that line our intestines, which promote gut health and decrease gut permeability. Short-chain fatty acids actually make serotonin, your "feel good" neurotransmitter that most antidepressants affect.

As discussed before, antibiotics are well known to cause a disruption in the microbiome. The microbes that survive a round of antibiotics are without competitors, which is why it's important to re-inoculate the digestive tract with beneficial microbes. We might provide a supplement to create the proper conditions that favor the growth of beneficial species and allow them to predominate; resisting species that might be harmful. This is especially important after an assault with an antibiotic when food wouldn't otherwise be sufficient.

There is a whole range of probiotics with different dosages, but in general there are two classes – Bifidobacterium and Lactobacillus. Lactobacillus is acquired through the transition from the mother's womb vaginally and Bifidobacterium is obtained through breast milk. Researchers are finding the benefits of specific strains of probiotics to target specific symptoms. For example, research has shown lactobacillus rhamnosus can increase the body's own production of gamma aminobutyric acid (GABA) and potentially treat anxiety.

In general, lactobacillus supports the immune system and digestion in the small intestine and Bifidobacterium resides in the large intestine to produce short-chain fatty acids that feed the enterocytes, cells of the large intestine.

It is important to get a probiotic that is broad-spectrum, pharmaceutical grade, and high-quality, preferably without fillers. Always check the expiration date before you buy them and, depending on the season, if you have them shipped, you'll want them shipped on ice. In other words, do not get them from box stores. The ones in the refrigerator are the most potent, but if you have the tendency to forget what's in the refrigerator or it's not compatible with your routine, getting a non-refrigerated one is fine. You'll want to keep the probiotics in a dark, cool place and use the bottle up quickly so that they don't go bad. They have to survive the manufacturing process, shelf life, and getting through your stomach to the intestine where they are needed.

Start at 20 to 30 billion CFU daily on an empty stomach, preferably at night, for general maintenance for 2 to 3 months; let's say if you had a round of antibiotics. Antibiotics can alter and disrupt the microbiota for twelve months.

I increase probiotics to progressively higher doses every month as tolerated to SHIFT the gut microbiome physiology, but the dose is dependent on the condition I am treating. I might add other types of probiotics like Saccharomyces boulardii, which is a good yeast that lowers the pH and decreases the likelihood for unwelcome types of yeast to take root. It's also great for handling traveler's diarrhea, as it prevents unwanted bacteria from attaching to the walls of your intestines and gets flushed out of your body.

Another type of probiotic is soil-based organisms that are spore-forming. They form a small spore making them resistant to heat, acid, and most antibiotics. They are more likely to survive stomach acid and reach the large intestine compared to other commonly used probiotic strains. These tend to do a better job of repairing the gut lining.

Some probiotics come with prebiotics to feed the probiotics. Some people don't tolerate prebiotics because they can cause gas and bloating. I tend to choose probiotics without prebiotics because people can choose prebiotic foods that they tolerate instead. Ultimately food is medicine, and we want to maintain the balance of the microbiome with natural probiotics in food once the physiology is shifted.

Most people tolerate probiotics well, but there are a few cases of people not tolerating them because they have SIBO (small intestinal bacterial overgrowth). They can change the consistency of bowel movement and affect transit time.

The next step is repairing the gut lining. You may feel really good after the first three steps and forget the fourth step, but this is extremely important because you will slip back to having symptoms if you don't make sure to do this step. Unfortunately, it's often forgotten, and people don't get to it because they either drop out of treatment or their focus is shifted to other things. It's this phase that seals the deal, it closes those gates and mans them. After addressing the root causes of increased gut permeability, like foods, infections, toxins, stress, and hormones, you need to close the gates and strengthen the army, your immune system, around those gates to prevent a relapse of symptoms. This is where maintenance comes in the next chapter.

Here's a trick question. If you looked at a donut, would you consider the hole to be part of the donut? Now imagine that donut turning into a tunnel or tube. Is that hole part of the tunnel? Add a mouth on one end and an anus on the other end. I'm trying to get you to see that the supposed "inside" of our gut, the tube between the mouth and the anus, is actually the "outside." This tube is called the lumen of the gut. Remember, the gut lining is one-cell layer thick. It has a mucus layer on top and the immune system below and the highway of the bloodstream below that. It doesn't take much to gain access to the body. In many ways, this is like flying into a foreign country. What does it take to get into the country from the moment you step off that plane to stepping into the taxi on the sidewalk? You have to get your passport out to tell them you belong here and if you didn't have a passport, you wouldn't get admitted. You have to go through customs to make sure you aren't carrying anything dangerous in your bags.

The cells that make up the lining of the small intestine, called enterocytes, is where we absorb the bulk of our nutrients. They form a barrier between the lumen of the intestines and the rest of the body. Their purpose is to regulate the absorption of nutrients and prevent bacteria, undigested food particles, or toxic substances from being absorbed into the bloodstream. In a healthy gut, about ninety percent of molecules are absorbed *through* the enterocytes, the transcellular pathway, processed as needed, and then passed on into the bloodstream.

However, some molecules, like water, can pass *between* the intestinal cells, the paracellular pathway, directly into the bloodstream. Enterocytes are held together by connections known as tight-junctions, adherens junctions, and desmosomes. The permeability of these junctions is managed by regulatory proteins and cytokines, which are affected by inflammatory foods and toxins, stress, and lipopolysaccharides from the cell wall of gram-negative bacteria resulting in "leaky gut." The regulatory proteins are zonulin, occludin and actomyosin; these can be measured to indirectly determine the level of gut permeability but not the cause. The scientific term for leaky gut is "increased intestinal permeability." When the gut is "leaky," it allows molecules that are normally kept out to pass through the lining of the intestines and into the bloodstream. That's like taking all of the police and customs officers out of the airport. When these factors cause tight junctions to stay open for too long, substances that otherwise wouldn't be allowed to cross the intestinal barrier are able to cross, then triggering an inflammatory immune response. Larger food particles that aren't recognized by the immune system end up being tagged for antibody processing and this causes the development of food sensitivities. All of these types of factors cause inflammation and when our bodies are exposed to inflammation over a long period of time, we tend to develop a variety of chronic diseases. There are strict rules about bringing certain things (like meats and food) into the country and the reason is that these can cause diseases in our flora and fauna. The gut has similar rules for similar reasons.

So, how do you repair the gut lining? Well, you can do this with food. Remember Grandma's chicken soup? Well, the main ingredient is bone broth, which contains the non-essential amino acids glutamine, glycine, proline, and alanine. Non-essential means that the body can make them, and it is not "essential" that they are provided through the diet. It prevents muscle wasting and heals injuries, wounds, burns, ulcers, and a damaged gut lining.

One can make bone broth easily at home. L-glutamine is the prime ingredient in any good formula. It's important to get a minimum of five grams three times a day – some people might need fifteen grams three times a day. This is only achievable and affordable using a powder. Other ingredients are aloe vera extract, deglycyrrhizinated licorice, arabinogalactan, slippery elm, N-acetyl, D-glucosamine, gamma oryzanol, cranesbill root, ginger root, marigold flower, quercetin, collagen powder, and marshmallow root. Taking fish oil is also an option. You can get various combinations of the above ingredients through supplements. They are best taken three times a day, ideally on an empty stomach for two to three months.

There is a very small percentage of people who react to glutamine as it gets converted into glutamate due to these people having certain SNPs. MSG, or monosodium glutamate, is well known to cause similar problems in the body as it stimulates the brain and can cause migraine headaches, attention problems, anxiety, and mood changes. If you have a reaction to MSG, you might react to L-glutamine. However, for the most part, people tolerate it well and thrive. If you have symptoms of itchiness, skin rash, hives, stomach upset, migraine headache, or a runny nose, that is usually a histamine reaction which can occur with bone broth. A histamine reaction is different from histamine intolerance. Some people confuse the two. This is where it's important to work with someone who knows what they are doing to help you navigate these waters.

Have you done the burp test yet?

Well, depending on the results, not only will apple cider vinegar (ACV) improve your digestion, but it is also very good for gut healing. Always buy apple cider vinegar with the "mother" (other words to look for: organic, raw, unfiltered) and dilute it before using it because it is too acidic to be taken straight. Mix one tablespoon with eight ounces of water. If the taste is too strong, dilute it some more. If you eat a lot of salads, then use this vinegar in place of others.

In summary, a properly functioning digestive system is critical to good health. In fact, problems with the gastrointestinal (GI) tract can cause more than just stomachaches, gas, bloating, or diarrhea. GI issues may underlie chronic health problems that seem unrelated to digestive health, including autoimmune diseases such as rheumatoid arthritis and Type 1 diabetes, skin problems such as eczema, acne, rosacea, and heart disease (just to name a few). In the bigger picture, how can we deal with all that can go wrong "down there"? In functional medicine we use a program that goes by the acronym of the Five Rs: remove, replace, re-inoculate, repair, and rebalance. When applied to various chronic health issues, the Five R program can lead to dramatic improvement in symptoms, and sometimes even complete resolution. The elements of the Five R program are described briefly below.

1. Remove

Remove stressors: get rid of things that negatively affect the environment of the GI tract including allergic foods, parasites, and potential problematic bacteria or yeast.

This might involve using an allergy "elimination diet" to find out what foods are causing GI symptoms or it may involve taking medications or herbs to eradicate a particular bug.

2. Replace

Replace digestive secretions: add back things like digestive enzymes, hydrochloric acid, and bile acids that are required for proper digestion and that may be compromised by diet, medications, diseases, aging, or other factors.

3. Re-inoculate

Help beneficial bacteria flourish by ingesting probiotic foods or supplements that contain the "good" GI bacteria such as *bifidobacteria* and *lactobacillus* species, and by consuming the high-soluble fiber foods that good bugs like to eat, called prebiotics.

4. Repair

Help the lining of the GI tract repair itself by supplying key nutrients that can often be in short supply in a compromised gut, such as zinc, antioxidants (e.g., vitamins A, C, and E), fish oil, and the amino acid glutamine.

5. Rebalance

It is important to pay attention to lifestyle choices. Sleep, exercise, and stress can all affect the GI tract. Balancing those activities is important to an optimal digestive tract.

Note: Used with permission from The Institute for Functional Medicine (IFM), the global leader in Functional Medicine and a collaborator in the transformation of healthcare. IFM is a 501(c)(3) nonprofit organization that believes Functional Medicine can help every individual reach their full potential for health and well-being. Under no circumstances may the whole or any part of the materials be translated into another language, nor may you create derivative or other works without IFM's prior written permission (for permission please contact info@ifm.org).

CHAPTER 13

Consolidating Gains

Now that you are feeling great, look at how much you accomplished in three months and pat yourself on the back. You probably didn't realize you could do *so* much in such a short time. Three months! Think about how you were then and how you are now. Amazing, right?

The rebalance phase is to establish certain habits into your life to maintain your results, but that requires reflection of what's changed and what created that change. Everyone is different. You need to do your own survey of yourself to figure it out for you.

Keep that journal in a special place. It will be a good reference to help you remember what worked and what didn't work. What you want to do is to maintain what you've accomplished. It might be hard to maintain because you are investing time into all of the steps, but you've got a life to get back to *or* life just happens and the things you do to stay well go by the wayside. What happens to most people is that they get called away to do something, like go on a business trip, or have a deadline they have to meet so everything stops, and all their energy goes to meet the deadline. It might be simply going on vacation and just not wanting to pack up those supplements. Let's face it, it's *work*! And sometimes something happens that gets you out of your routine.

Expect that this is going to happen, and when it happens, *take notes*! Pay attention. Please, don't beat yourself up- *that* is a complete waste of time. I will tell you right now, do not think that going back to the way you did things before you read this book will maintain your results. It will take work to keep your results. Why would you want to, anyway? You felt horrible!

It's important to reflect on what the changes are that made the biggest impact. Look at your MSQ score that you've been doing monthly or the notes you've been taking to see which intervention gave you the most results. You need to continue these one or two things at all costs. When that "thing" happens that pulls you away from your routine, you will need to find ways to continue those items in your routine that got you well.

I want to let you know that you need to pay attention now for certain symptoms starting up again. These are your red flags. The moment you experience them, you need to stop and pay attention and review what you've been doing over the last week.

What healthy habits dropped off?

What did you add back into your diet purposely or accidentally in the last forty-eight hours? Open up a page in your journal, write the date, and do a brain dump of everything you ate. Is anything new? Put a circle around the new ones. Close your eyes and ask your *body*, not your brain, what food it thought might not have agreed with it. Write that down. Some people think this is silly to think about, but your body knows. Have you ever eaten out and had a meal with ten to fifteen ingredients in it, and got sick; throwing up and having diarrhea, but you *knew* that it was a certain ingredient in the meal? And from that day on, you haven't had that ingredient again because your body just says *no*! Well, there you go.

Let's SHIFT through what works. Ask yourself, "Is this a must for me?"

Stress

A program for movement or exercise. How do you feel *after* you do this? Have you missed a day of yoga and wished you hadn't? Some people need to have a daily practice. Stress is something you can't necessarily plan for as it can blindside you, but you can have a prepared response for when it happens. Having a response to stress allows you to feel in control. Create a space that feels safe to you, do that hand massage, take that bath with Epsom salt, listen to new age music, and pull out that yoga mat and get into child pose. Pull out your favorite blanket and have that cup of tea. Nurture yourself. It is not a selfish thing to do. It's recharging your batteries. Stress is often overlooked and hard to manage. It sneaks its way in and you don't realize it until it's too late. That's why having a comfort zone and basket prepared and ready for those times will help you. No feeling guilty allowed. I'm telling you that you need this.

Hormones

Initially the primary hormone of concern is cortisol, which is the body's response to adrenalin. When chronic inflammation declines, cortisol declines. Adrenal hormones do a dance with the thyroid hormones to keep the body in homeostasis. The return to homeostasis of the sex hormones is dependent on your stage of life. Other hormones like Vitamin D and melatonin decline under stress, and insulin and leptin increase under stress. Hormones play a critical role in inter-communication and regulation of systems.

Infections

If you had a gut dysbiosis that was shifted into balance with the Five Rs, took supplements, and felt better, generally, you should be able to discontinue the supplements. Stop them one at a time, noting the date and how you feel. Write down what symptoms you had prior to starting them to remind you. Life stressors, going on a trip, and eating something bad or choosing to eat something you fully know will cause your symptoms because it's your wedding could all increase that gut permeability. You can decrease gut permeability if you restart the supplements even for a couple of days. Taking the supplements to repair the gut lining or taking probiotics for a week may bring you back into balance. You can learn how to decide when to use supplements to manage your symptoms. Just know, it's not all lost.

Foods

You may be eating a restricted food plan and haven't ventured into putting foods back into your diet. Some people become fearful that they will get sick again and sometimes are satisfied just eating the diet the way it is. The problem with this is that it is not sustainable and puts you at risk of not having many choices and eating the same foods every day. Therefore, you end up not enjoying food or eating foods you shouldn't be eating. This is a set up for failure.

The microbiome thrives with a variety of foods and it's best to rotate your foods every seventy-two hours. Introduce foods after the repair phase. Start eating foods that contain fiber, which feeds the good bacteria that produces short-chain fatty acids, which are the main source of energy that strengthen the enterocytes, cells lining your colon. Here is a list to start: lentils, black beans, pinto beans, kidney beans, navy beans, edamame, nuts, and chia seeds. Start eating foods that are fermented to feed the gut microbiome. Chapter 9 has a list of fermented foods to try. Write down the symptoms you will be scanning your mind and body for each day and see what comes up for you.

Sometimes, one can experience symptoms up to seven days later, especially mental health symptoms. If you are going to add a food group in, do it at the beginning of the weekend and listen to your body. For most people who have a return of symptoms, these symptoms occur within forty-eight hours. Write down all of the foods you want to add back in on a list, starting with your favorites (except gluten and dairy). Be methodical about it. Add one food or food group in for a day, then stop that food and track any change in symptoms. I would start with cooked foods first – vegetables, fruits, nuts, parts of the egg, non-GMO soy, and corn. If you really want dairy, start with aged cheeses as they have the least amount of casein, or fermented dairy like goat kefir, but stay away from fresh sources of dairy like milk, ice cream, sour cream, ricotta, or cottage cheese. If you have these foods, make a note of it and pay attention to any reaction. Use it as an opportunity to observe. No beating yourself up for having it is allowed!

Gluten is a tough one to add back in, especially if you noticed a big difference taking it out. Try eating some wonderful gluten-free bread. Make sure you don't have celiac disease. If anyone in your family has it, you might too. My husband had one gene and his aunt had celiac disease. I had one gene. I have non-celiac gluten sensitivity but our son has celiac disease because he got one gene from each of his parents. Start with sourdough bread, as the rising and fermentation process in this bread reduces the load of gluten. See how you feel. The thing about gluten is sometimes the quantity and chronicity of eating gluten is what creates the problem. I have found that some people are able to eat it once in a while. It is important to understand why you might not tolerate glutinous foods, as some people think that it is gluten that is the problem when it is actually eating grains in general. Too many grainy carbs can make a person feel very sick and think it's gluten, so if you are grain-free or light on grains, then try eating gluten-free grains first.

Once you figure out what you can and cannot eat, you will need to plan for vacations, for meals during the week, business trips, packing food for yourself, and having shelf-stable emergency foods for when your routine changes. I keep a supply of delicious gluten-free crackers in my car. When we eat out, I bring the box in with me and use my own crackers to eat with the cheese tray that I order as an appetizer and show these crackers to the restaurant owner with the hopes that they will provide them to everyone. I keep gluten-free protein bars in my car and at work if I haven't had time to prepare lunch. You need to have a game plan. Part of that game plan might be investing time on the weekend to meal prep for the week. Make lunches and dinners ahead of time. There are some wonderful recipes online for making salads in a jar and they are beautiful to look at as well.

Toxins

Get into the habit of reading the ingredients on all packaging of all products and ask questions about products. Removing toxins from your house or your life is a continuous process. When you go shopping, replace toxic products you have at home with less or non-toxic ones. There might be a product that you really liked that you eliminated earlier in this process, and now find you can add it back in and see how your immune system reacts. If it does react, you have some more work to do to heal your gut lining. You will want to work with someone who understands chemical sensitivities.

For some people, it's easier to just get rid of everything – give it away and start with a fresh pantry and kitchen closet full of new products – but some people can't afford to do that.

You might still be "in-process" on certain areas of your healing journey and that's okay. That's why it's called a journey.

Create a plan for the next few months for how you are going to continue this journey.

Your mindset is your friend. Having a practice of expressing joy and gratitude on a daily basis will always dial you into what's really important.

Remember, there really are no rules, only personal choices. Some people live by the word "should." "I should do..." My response to that is: "Says who?" When you really think about where that statement comes from, it's easier to discard. Right now, does X work for you or not? That is the question.

I say, "Never make any decision based on guilt, fear, shame, and anger. Do it because you want to!" This is my very own original quote. I've had long discussions about this in psychotherapy sessions with my patients and some repeat it back to me because once they get it, they see that it works. If you focus on the things you want and you have all of these feelings coming up around them, take note of those feelings and do something about the feelings separately. Don't let those feelings get in the way of what you want.

Approach life with curiosity and investigation. Be open and increase your awareness of your surroundings. Know that there is a reason for everything, and things happen for a reason. It may sound trite to you, but there is a deeper meaning to the statement. It may not have come into your conscious awareness.

Change your day-to-day mindset by planning for your one-year mark using your perfect-life vision. If you haven't done that yet, do it now. You need to work toward something, not function in a void. Some people do things because they were told to do them, because they need to do them, or because they should do them. These decisions are driven by fear, guilt, shame or anger, not by desire. It comes back around to this: what do you want? Ask yourself what is it that you *want*. This is a scary question for people because it conjures up feelings of selfishness that are confused with feelings of self-nurture and self-affirmation.

Everyone needs to have a purposeful life. What do you *want*? Creating habits and simplifying your life will reduce your stress. What can you cut out of your life that offers little return? Changing habits is scary and hard, but maintaining the changes is harder. The key to making these changes last in the long run is making sure that it feels right to you, that you are doing them for the right reason, actually for *you*, and most importantly, that you're having fun.

CHAPTER 14

Avoiding Derailments

You picked up this book for a reason. There is a part of you that is railing against what everyone else is telling you and you're just looking for answers. "Why the heck am I feeling this way?" "I know how I feel and it's not good and I know this isn't depression, but I don't know what this is." I hope that this book has given you some insight as to what is going on and why.

Now the decision you need to make is what to do about it. The first thing that happens is a feeling of being overwhelmed. You don't like where you are, Point A, and you want to be at Point B. Sit with that feeling and write down everything that comes to mind that is preventing you getting from Point A to Point B. Well, where is Point B anyway? Go back to the Perfect Life Vision exercise in Chapter 6, remind yourself of where that is, and imagine the possibilities.

Once you decide what you want to change or where you want to be in life, even if it's in the short-term (and you can have short-term goals and long-term goals), then you want to check in with yourself and think about where the resistance is.

Resistance is a psychotherapy term. Doing psychotherapy is easy for me. It comes naturally. I put myself in a place of compassion and meet the patient where they are suffering, sense the first layer of resistance, and gently point it out to them because much of the time, they generally aren't aware of it. Whether or not they are aware of it, there are "parts" of the resistance that they don't see and then that is what we address. After these resistances are brought to the forefront, they have a choice, to continue in the same direction or move into a new direction. In the end, the person learns this approach to help themselves without me.

People resist without being in therapy. Resistance arises out of our defensive style and our personalities. Like any defense, it protects us from something that hurts. Examples of psychological resistance may include perfectionism, procrastination, preoccupations, distractions, avoidance, isolation, a need to be seen as independent or invulnerable, an inability to accept compliments or constructive criticism, erroneous belief systems, and even apathy.

Simply stated, resistance is how we protect ourselves from awareness of the things that might overwhelm us. This does not happen consciously. This is why psychotherapy takes a long time. It's why self-help books are always coming out and don't work for everyone. These books can't adapt to your forms of resistance or to your personality. There will be times in our lives when we're open to new ideas that run up against our resistance. When we are not open to it, the best self-help book in the world won't reach us.

Patients describe resistance as feeling like a wall that pushes back. If you ever feel like you're grinding your gears, it's because of resistance. If you were in a rowboat rowing in one direction and the parts of you that are resisting were rowing in the other direction, you would not move. Resistance is at its highest when the issue is most sensitive and makes you feel vulnerable – it's too close to home.

I bring this up because for you to move forward, you need to see where you are resistant to change and address this with a coach or psychotherapist. These resistances can get in the way of more than just prioritizing your health.

Change can be hard when a person decides to take action and go down a new path. What they take with them along the journey are old behaviors. These old behaviors can cause a person to stumble on their journey. One behavior is destructive self-criticism, and it comes with an unkind impatience of oneself. Some people say the worst things to themselves - things they would never say to anyone else. There is an unconscious belief that harshness and whip-cracking keeps one motivated and gets results. There is plenty of research that demonstrates that this method does not work. Approaching changes in one's lifestyle with kindness, curiosity, and compassion gets results much faster. I advise my patients to say, "Whoops! That wasn't supposed to happen. I wonder why it did?" The attempt to change behavior deserves praise. Pat yourself on the back! Examination of the process allows for a micro-change in method while you cheerlead yourself, providing support to try it again. You might think this is silly, but it works better than what you are likely doing, and you learn something about yourself each and every time.

Some people think that they are selfish for doing things for themselves, thinking it's "pampering," and confuse it with providing self-care. Self-care is essential maintenance. Keeping up on your automobile care by changing the oil, lube, filter, and having the tires checked or rotated increases the life and value of your car. Keeping up on your home care protects your investment as well. Mowing the lawn, painting the house inside and out, changing the filters and checking for leaks and mold are all part of maintenance.

None of what we do for our car and home is paid for by car and home insurance. Yet, some people think that our health insurance plans should pay for our own health maintenance. If you didn't care for your house by maintaining the roof, eventually it would leak and cause a great deal of damage. Even at its worst, if you were negligent in caring for your home and making it unsafe to live in, your home insurance wouldn't necessarily kick in. Running your car into the ground or not fixing those scratches eventually leads to the car dying or rusting, and your auto insurance wouldn't necessarily pay for those things. It would have to be catastrophic, like a tree falling on the house and two cars colliding on the road, for the insurance to kick in. Our lifestyles and bad habits are what is causing us to rust, mold, and leak. You can always get a new car or move to a new house, but you can't get a new body. Fortunately, the body is equipped to relatively quickly heal itself, when given the raw materials, removed barriers, and the investment of time.

Some people feel like they don't have the money or the time to invest in themselves. Doing this work is an investment and you have to feel that you deserve it, but also expect that you will likely feel better, be more productive, and live a longer life because of it.

It comes down to priorities. Some people have no problem buying a $1,000 cell phone and paying $200 monthly for a phone plan and $200 monthly for cable TV because it's a "necessity." Some people spend money on dyeing their hair, doing their nails, smoking cigarettes, and drinking alcohol treating these as necessities. Then there is all of the money spent on conveniences of buying coffee daily or eating lunch and/or dinner out. If you really looked at where your money is going and look at what can be discontinued in service to your health, you might find that you actually save money. For example, you will find that you won't need to buy skin creams because your skin is no longer dry, deodorant because you no longer have body odor, acne creams because your skin is clearer, makeup and antiwrinkle products because you look naturally younger. You may not need to buy as much coffee because you have natural energy, sunscreen because you don't burn as easily, mosquito repellent because you don't attract those mosquitoes anymore. You won't be spending a fortune on over-the-counter medications like antihistamines, antacids, laxatives, and pain medications.

Time is not found; time is made. Think about how you actually spend your time. Think about the web surfing you do and the Facebook and Instagram postings and emails you read. There are ways to find this time. Finding the answers to why you feel the way you do takes time because there can be multiple layers that need to come to your awareness first. Progress requires effort with a knowing that you will get to the other side of your goals.

Looking at all of your resistances, obstacles, priorities and objections is really all part of the journey. What are your obstacles to change and getting your life back?

Some people get overwhelmed with everything they think they need to do and don't know where to start. I'm sure reading this book started to help you think of all of the areas you need to address. The beauty of functional medicine is that you can start anywhere. Just pick any one area that feels like the right place for you to start. What is manageable right now? You can add another layer when you are ready. There is no one right path. If you don't know where to start, start with food.

Lastly, many people don't move forward with this kind of work because of lack of support from their doctors, friends, or family. Fortunately, functional medicine is on the rise and increasing numbers of people are aware of its power. People have heard of gluten-free and see changes in products at their grocery stores. There is a whole movement of people creating CSAs and farmer's markets and planting their own gardens.

It takes courage to believe in yourself and get what you need to feel better. There is a growing community of people who can support you. It's just about finding it locally. You can look for a provider through the Physician Locator on the Institute for Functional Medicine website www.ifm.org. I'm on there.

Regaining your mental and physical health is a journey. Just like in every journey, there are many twists and turns. Sometimes it can be scary and other times, exhilarating. In the process, you learn something about yourself, meet new friends, grow emotionally, and gain a different and brighter outlook. The process can be hard at times and you might want to give up. If you stay on track by treading with patience, empathy, curiosity, and kindness to yourself, you will be successful.

CHAPTER 15

What's Next?

"Follow your inner moonlight;
don't hide the madness."
– Allen Ginsberg

Well, I hope you have a better understanding of what is *really* going on in your mind and body, a decrease in your emotional symptoms, an improvement in your sleep and energy. Most importantly, I hope you feel validated and empowered, and that you have gained some control of your life! I hope you understand a different model of thinking and that mental illness is not a disease. Diagnoses of depression are names given to a cluster of symptoms for the purposes of doing research, submitting insurance claims, and prescribing medications.

Many people have come to my office with horrific stories of being involuntarily hospitalized on a psych unit because they are frustrated and exhausted with trying to find answers that they become desperate and even suicidal. They feel afraid, invalidated, and are made to feel crazy or even labeled with hypochondriasis. All they know is that they don't feel well and don't know why, and they just want a solution. Instead, after going to numerous doctors, they are only told that their exam and bloodwork is normal and referred to specialists who tell them the same or who find "something" which takes them down another rabbit hole. It's like being Alice in Wonderland, but it's Nightmare-ville instead. The message they consistently get is that it's all in their head.

They eventually hear about functional medicine, find me, and feel heard, validated, and ultimately empowered in their health. Sometimes they do, indeed, need some assistance with medication while they search for the root causes of their problems. They bring the body back into balance and eventually come off medication. Conventional medications ought to be used in the shortest term possible.

I promised that I would tell you what I think happened to my mother. I believe her perfect storm was living in a new country, isolated, not speaking the language, having the stress of raising two young babies. And then being hit by a car and suffering from a head injury resulted in her symptoms of psychosis. Having two more babies stressed her body enormously such that she declined further. We all started to eat processed foods like packaged macaroni and cheese, pizza, and drank soda, which triggered her rheumatoid arthritis. When we went to India, she ate food that her genes recognized. Most Indian food is gluten-free, full of fruits and vegetables, and includes locally produced wheat and dairy. When she returned to the US, she resumed eating processed foods and had a relapse in her symptoms. I'm sure there are details I don't know, but I am satisfied with that explanation.

I hope this book has helped you to understand why a doctor would draw the conclusion that you are depressed. It's my wish that you now understand what depression is, and how to decide if and when an antidepressant is an appropriate solution for you. Hopefully, you've learned a different model of thinking, whether it is depression or not.

I hope you have learned what is *actually* going on by doing some assessments and drawing a timeline of events. You have identified when various elements came together and developed into the perfect storm(s) in your life causing your immune system to wane or even crash.

I hope you've learned about the root causes of inflammation and how this affects the immune system, how to put out the fire, so to speak, and rebuild the immune system starting with optimizing digestion; shifting your physiology by Removing infections, stress, and toxins and unhealthy foods, Replacing the missing nutrients with healthy foods, Reinoculating the microbiome; and Repairing the gut lining. I hope you've learned what you personally need to do to Rebalance or maintain your newfound mental and physical health and are informed as to where to get more information.

I hope you understand that it's possible to resolve your depression, anxiety, and concomitant symptoms with food and lifestyle changes but most importantly by healing your gut. It's work but it's do-able and there is, indeed, another way if you find that medications aren't working, don't want to take medications and/or have side effects from medications.

Despite the knowledge you've acquired from this book, success will require putting yourself first, believing you are worth it, investing time and energy to change habits and surroundings, and connecting with people you love. When you honor yourself, the people around you, the rhythms of life and the universe, you see that everything is connected not only on the inside but the outside as well. You come full circle.

Acknowledgments

The idea of writing a book was triggered in my head when I had a tarot card reading with Maribeth McNair, The Happy Medium. She told me I'd write a book and I said, "No way! I can't even imagine such a thing!" as I absolutely hate to write. Thank you for planting the seed.

It took a year, maybe two, before I seriously considered this possibility because I became frustrated with the current medical system and I realized I had a unique persepctive on assessment and treatment of conditions connected to emotional problems. I started to work with Lynda Goldman of *Wellness Ink*, who led a group of "authors-to-be" to learn about the process of writing a book. I met a lot of wonderful people. I wrote a few chapters. Thank you for letting me know that I am worthy and that writing a book is possible.

I found Angela Lauria of *Author Incubator* through one of my best friends. I was hooked after watching her webinar. I completed an application and was accepted in weeks. I thank Angela and her entire team – especially Ramses Rodriguez for persistently being in my face and Bethany Davis for giving me the courage when I was terrified – for transforming me into the author that wrote this book in nine weeks. You are right, Angela! Writing the book is the easy part. It's not perfect, but my message is out there. If I waited for perfection, it would not have been written.

I mentioned one of my best friends above. That would be Rajka Milanovic, M.D. We talk weekly and support each other emotionally. I met her at Visions Healthcare, Inc. the day she started, and I knew she was my soul sister. I want to thank Kat Toups, M.D. for her insights and believing in me with just a "knowing," if you know what I mean. She will soon be publishing her book, *Demystifiyng Dementia*. Look out! There are many friends and colleagues who have been supportive of me, but these two have especially sustained me in the process of writing.

I can't thank Edward Levitan, M.D. enough for giving me the opportunity to shadow him. He introduced me to the world of functional medicine. I have been paying it forward by letting other doctors and nurses shadow me. While I have been on this journey, I have networked with hundreds of other functional medicine practitioners and have the joy of having a fantastic *business* (inside joke) partner, Sally Davidson, ANP. We teach each other all of the time. I am grateful to be her partner and a member of these groups.

My partner of forty years, Matt, has been my rock through-out my life and this process is no exception. He deserves an award for best husband, no doubt. To my three children – thank you for your patience and your unconditional love, but especially for giving me permission to talk about you and your experiences for the good of easing the suffering of others. It means a lot to me. I thank all of my extended family members for their support.

My office manager, Carol Carpenter, is my rock at work. She is humble, works quietly in the background, but always makes sure that I am comfortable, have everything I need and is my personal cheerleader – kind of like the mom I always wanted. She deserves an award, too.

Last but not least, I am very grateful for the support of my patients. Without you, none of this would have been possible. I learn from you as much as you learn from me. You keep me on my toes and are not afraid to challenge me. Because of you, I walk the walk, not just talk the talk. Thank you for teaching me. You are my Watsons. We are a team.

Let's keep dancing. I love you all.
Achina

Thank You

Thank you so much for reading *What If It's* Not *Depression? Your Guide to Answers and Solutions.* If you've made it this far, I know one or two things about you. First, you're more ready than ever to start your health journey and get your life back! And second, maybe you also start at the end of the book before diving in (ha! me too!).

I would love to learn about you, your journey, and your success in pursuing *your* mental health goals and getting your life back. Please keep in touch! I'm most active on my personal Facebook page. To continue the conversation, email me at AStein@HealthySelfBootCamp.com or request a free consultation.

As a thank you, I have created a free masterclass to introduce you to my new online health-coaching program. It's a companion program to this book to assist people to sort out whether they are depressed and to reach their mental and physical health goals. If you are interested in working with me, email me or go to the website to register for a free consultation.

Email: AStein@HealthySelfBootCamp.com

Webpage: www.fxnmind.com

About the Author

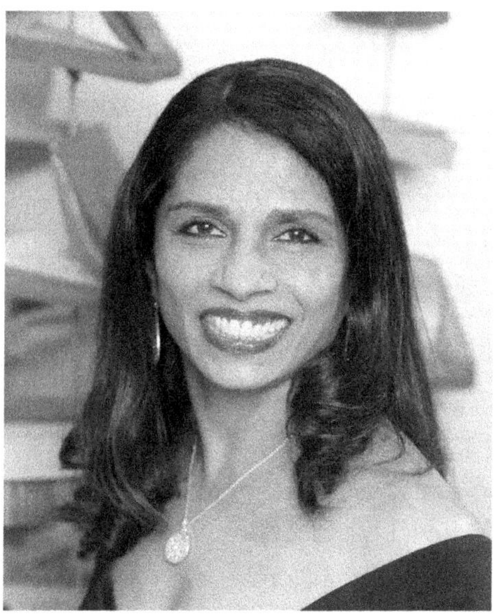

Dr. Achina Stein is an osteopathic physician who graduated from the UMDNJ school of osteopathic medicine (now called Rowan University School of Osteopathic Medicine) in 1990 and has been in practice as a board-certified psychiatrist for twenty-five-plus years. Her osteopathic roots set her apart from conventional psychiatrists because of her use of osteopathic philosophy, manual medicine, and biopsychosocial treatment approach.

Initially on a psychoanalytic track, she became well trained in psychodynamic psychotherapy and CBT and does psychotherapy with a number of patients with underlying trauma issues, specifically mood and dissociative disorders.

She has much experience using psychopharmacology working with the prison population, community mental health centers with the chronic and persistent mental health population, and geriatric psychiatry inpatient population. She understood the limitations of treatment with medication and continually searched for other modalities of treatment.

Propelled by her son's health crisis in 2010, she found functional medicine, which resolved all of his health problems as well as her own. Since 2012, she has become trained in and practices functional medicine. She was certified by the American Board of Integrative and Holistic Medicine and is a certified practitioner of the Institute for Functional Medicine.

Dr. Stein is a Distinguished Fellow of the American Psychiatric Association and awarded the Exemplary Psychiatrist Award by NAMI-RI in 2008.

She is presently in private practice in RI and co-owner of Functional Mind, LLC with advanced nurse practitioner Sally Davidson. www.fxnmind.com

She has lived in Rhode Island since 2000 with her husband and has three adult children. She enjoys playing ultimate frisbee, growing her own vegetables, dancing, and singing.

Appendix A:
Lab Work and
Specialty Testing

List of blood work typically obtained by me and other functional medicine practitioners.

You can order them yourself – just google "buy lab test online." There are companies available such as the following where you do not need to have a doctor's orders. Some include www.directlabs.com and www.labtestsonline.org. I have an account with www.truehealthlabs.com. There are more and more available to you. Even Quest Diagnostics is offering labs without need for a physician or nurse practitioner to provide you a lab slip. You can take your health into your own hands.

The labs I typically order right from the beginning are:

- CBC – complete blood count
- CMP- comprehensive metabolic panel – fasting
- Thyroid panel – freeT3, freeT4, Total T3, TSH – high sensitivity, reverse T3, anti TPO Ab, anti TG Ab
- Vitamin D, 25 hydroxy

- Vitamin B12 and methylmalonic acid
- RBC folate
- RBC magnesium
- RBC zinc,
- Plasma selenium
- Plasma copper
- C reactive protein, high sensitivity
- DHEA sulfate
- Iron panel – serum iron, serum ferritin, TIBC, transferrin iron saturation %, serum transferrin receptor
- Lipid panel with calculated LDL
- VAP panel – breakdown LDL and HDL
- HgbA1c, fasting
- Insulin, serum, fasting
- Carnitine – free, total, esters
- Coenzyme Q10, serum
- Candida IgG, IgM, IgA
- EBV titers – all 4 values – Nuclear Ab, Viral capsid Ab IgG, Viral capsid Ab IgM, Early Antigen D Ab IgG.
- Free and total testosterone – if getting testosterone injection, get blood levels on day two because that is when it peaks. Want it > 500. Younger person >900
- Progesterone – day 20 if still menstruating
- Estradiol
- Urinalysis with reflex culture
- Heavy metals: Lead, Mercury, Cadmium, Arsenic

Specialty Testing

- Stool test – Diagnostic Solutions Lab – GIMAP
- Organic Acid Testing – Great Plains Lab
- IgG Food sensitivity testing – Dunwoody Labs is

preferable; Alletess in past.

- Salivary cortisol levels – Adrenal Stress Index – Genova, Doctor's Data or you may combine sex hormone testing with this through DUTCH

Other Testing – If Suspicious or if Symptoms Are Not Getting Better

- Lyme disease and co-infections panel – Igenex or Vibrant Wellness
- Mold panel – Great Plains Lab
- Autoimmune panel – Vibrant Wellness or Cyrex Labs
- Viral panel – Vibrant Wellness
- PANNS – Strep, Staph and Mycoplasma
- 3-hour SIBO test

www.ingramcontent.com/pod-product-compliance
Lightning Source LLC
Chambersburg PA
CBHW061525120726

48001CB00004B/1406